WHAT DOCTORS DON'T TELL YOU

HEART
DISEASE

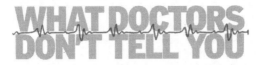

HEART DISEASE

Drug-Free
Alternatives to
Prevent and Reverse
Heart Disease

Editor
Lynne McTaggart

HAY HOUSE

Carlsbad, California • New York City • London • Sydney
Johannesburg • Vancouver • Hong Kong • New Delhi

First published and distributed in the United Kingdom by:
Hay House UK Ltd, Astley House, 33 Notting Hill Gate, London W11 3JQ
Tel: +44 (0)20 3675 2450; Fax: +44 (0)20 3675 2451; www.hayhouse.co.uk

Published and distributed in the United States of America by:
Hay House Inc., PO Box 5100, Carlsbad, CA 92018-5100
Tel: (1) 760 431 7695 or (800) 654 5126
Fax: (1) 760 431 6948 or (800) 650 5115; www.hayhouse.com

Published and distributed in Australia by:
Hay House Australia Ltd, 18/36 Ralph St, Alexandria NSW 2015
Tel: (61) 2 9669 4299; Fax: (61) 2 9669 4144; www.hayhouse.com.au

Published and distributed in the Republic of South Africa by:
Hay House SA (Pty) Ltd, PO Box 990, Witkoppen 2068
info@hayhouse.co.za; www.hayhouse.co.za

Published and distributed in India by:
Hay House Publishers India, Muskaan Complex, Plot No.3, B-2,
Vasant Kunj, New Delhi 110 070
Tel: (91) 11 4176 1620; Fax: (91) 11 4176 1630; www.hayhouse.co.in

Distributed in Canada by:
Raincoast Books, 2440 Viking Way, Richmond, B.C. V6V 1N2
Tel: (1) 604 448 7100; Fax: (1) 604 270 7161; www.raincoast.com

Text © WDDTY Publishing Ltd., 2016

While every care was taken in preparing this material, neither the
authors nor the publisher can accept any responsibility for any damage
or harm caused by any treatment, advice or information contained in
this publication, or for any material on third party websites. You should
consult a qualified practitioner before undertaking any treatment.

A catalogue record for this book is available from the British Library.

ISBN: 978-1-78180-336-3

Printed and bound by CPI Group (UK) Ltd, Croydon, CR0 4YY

For our readers

CONTENTS

Part III: Alternative Solutions

ABOUT WHAT DOCTORS DON'T TELL YOU

What Doctors Don't Tell You is one of the world's most respected information resources about safe and effective treatments in alternative medicine and the dangers and limitations of much of conventional medicine.

WDDTY, as it's popularly known, is a monthly glossy magazine, an award-winning website (www.wddty.com) and a community of people around the world seeking out safer and effective therapies.

Its hallmark is health information backed by exhaustive scientific research; in fact, readers have come to place such trust in the accuracy of WDDTY that information in its pages has even been cited in courts of law.

WDDTY's research has helped many thousands of people overcome a vast variety of conditions and regain their health, while many more have maintained their health, thanks to WDDTY's broad reach of research, which also encompasses nutrition, exercise and other lifestyle issues.

It was started in 1989 by its two editors, Lynne McTaggart, bestselling author of *The Field*, *The Intention Experiment* and *The Bond*, and her husband, Bryan Hubbard, a former *Financial Times* journalist and author of *The Untrue Story of You*.

McTaggart and Hubbard launched their publication in 1989 out of a sense of frustration with conventional medicine, and a desire to tell others about its shortcomings, after an odyssey of Lynne's to solve her own puzzling health problem. When nothing – from conventional or alternative medicine – seemed to help, she began doing her own research into what appeared to be the most appropriate therapy and sought out the doctor, a nutritional pioneer, most likely to help her. In the process, she realized that patients were more likely to get better if they were put in charge of their own decision-making.

Lynne's eyes had first been opened to the limitation of conventional medicine by one of America's leading doctors. Before creating What Doctors Don't Tell You, Lynne, as editor of a national newspaper syndicate, launched the national column of the legendary Dr Robert Mendelsohn, one of the first doctors to blow the whistle on medical practices.

WDDTY began life in 1989 as an eight-page newsletter and has evolved into a glossy international magazine that has attracted many thousands of readers and subscribers. It is currently published in the UK and the US, and under licence in 12 other countries.

Its editorial panel include 12 noted pioneers of nutritional, environmental and alternative medicine, nine of whom are medical doctors.

The launch of WDDTY in the UK soon got the press's attention. *The Times* called it 'a voice in the silence,' while *The Observer* said it 'rang the alarm bells on procedures long before they became the stuff of national panic.'

WDDTY has also published 20 books on health conditions, and has several audio courses available.

The What Doctors Don't Tell You website has twice won Most Popular Health Website of the Year award, landing more votes than such well-known sites as BUPA and the National Health Service. It attracts hundreds of thousands of visitors every month, who use its searchable 10,000-page database for vital information about overcoming virtually every condition without drugs or surgery.

In 2015, WDDTY Publishing Ltd was awarded Ethical Business of the Year by popular reader vote, in a competition conducted by the magazine *Kindred Spirit*.

Over the years WDDTY has been acknowledged as one of the world's very best health resources by several commentators, including leading publisher and health campaigner Burton Goldberg, leading holistic healer Dr John Diamond, the Holistic Health Library and UK allergy specialist Dr John Mansfield.

To find out more and to subscribe to the magazine, visit www.wddty.com.

INTRODUCTION

The number of deaths from heart disease reads like a terrifying indictment of our modern lives and, indeed, our modern medicine. Although cancer, stroke and even iatrogenic (medically induced) illness are close runners-up, heart disease is still the number one killer in the West. A decade ago, one million people died of heart disease in the USA and 160,000 in the UK. Despite claims of tremendous strides made in cardiac treatment, supposedly sophisticated breakthroughs in prevention and a great deal of self-congratulation, today's statistics tell a very different story – of nothing less than a modern medical failure.

Cardiovascular disease kills one person every 37 seconds in the USA alone. In fact, cardiovascular disease – an umbrella term that includes coronary heart disease, myocardial infarction (heart attack), angina, heart failure and stroke – is still responsible for nearly one third of all deaths. Atherosclerosis – the narrowing of the arteries – is a major cause of heart disease and continues its relentless rise.

The UK and US governments, the food and pharmaceutical industries, the medical profession and a host of manufacturers of the latest treatment solutions have spawned entire industries in an attempt to make a dent in these sobering statistics. These include:

⇨ Widely disseminating the benefits of a low-fat diet

⇨ Developing a food and pharmaceutical monolith devoted entirely to heart disease prevention

⇨ Producing a coterie of ever more sophisticated drugs and surgical procedures

⇨ Making universal recommendations to take aspirin and statins as just-in-case measures.

However, the bald fact remains that, despite every one of these efforts, heart disease continues to kill more Westerners than any other ailment. The incidence of heart disease fell in the USA between 1979 and 1989 by 30 per cent, but researchers had no explanation for these statistics except for the reduction in smoking. Although medicine has helped more heart attack patients avoid a second attack, it's done little to stop deaths following the first attack. Of the 1.5 million people who have a heart attack in the USA each year, just 350,000 live to tell the tale: in other words, the first heart attack is often the last. In all, one-fifth – or 58.8 million – of Americans still suffer from cardiovascular disease. Moreover, heart disease in general – which includes high blood pressure and irregular heartbeat as well as blocked arteries – still accounts for 40 per cent of all deaths.

What is heart disease?

The term 'heart disease' is in fact a misnomer, as the problem is not so much the pumping organ itself but the arteries that feed it. If these become narrowed, blood flow to the heart is restricted, causing it to malfunction. The immediate cause of death is a 'sudden' heart attack, but this is the endpoint of the slow progression of coronary artery disease whereby, over decades, the arterial walls become furred up and finally blocked with fatty matter called plaque, thereby severely restricting blood flow to the heart and often causing angina, or pain in the chest. Over time, these plaques can harden, and blood clots form around them. If a clot completely blocks the artery, and too little oxygen via the blood reaches the heart, a portion of the heart's muscle will die, causing cardiac arrest, or heart attack.

The conventional medical view used to be that atherosclerosis was an inevitable result of ageing, but today heart disease is considered almost entirely the fault of the sufferer's lifestyle – with smoking, lack of exercise and, above all, a high-fat diet playing a major role.

The logic behind the 'fat causes atherosclerosis' theory, which forms the foundation of all medical treatment, is simple. Arteries become narrowed by deposits of cholesterol; fat in the diet contains cholesterol; so fat must cause atherosclerosis. The idea is so entrenched in the medical mind that the proposition is no longer a theory, but established fact.

The only problem is that the theory is manifestly wrong. As a consequence, so are most of the medical approaches to the epidemic.

From 1989 onwards, *What Doctors Don't Tell You* has been among the first publications to blow the whistle on much of heart disease prevention and treatment as largely misguided and unproven. In issue after issue, we reported on studies showing that lowering supposed risk factors like cholesterol levels doesn't do any good and, indeed, may actually do harm. Over the years, we've also covered non-drug treatments that show evidence of success.

To produce this book, we've pulled together the best of the evidence our publication has gathered over the years on alternative and conventional approaches to the most common heart problems. This includes coverage of atherosclerosis, angina, high blood pressure, heart flutters and irregular heartbeat (or atrial fibrillation), and stroke – which is essentially a 'heart attack' in the brain caused by a problem involving blood circulation, and so is often lumped together with heart disease.

As you'll discover in these pages, this book takes a very different approach to heart disease than you're likely to be given by your doctor. We've scoured the medical literature for evidence of what works and what doesn't in conventional and alternative medicine. As a consequence, we're unabashedly critical of the standard medical approach to preventing and treating heart attacks, high cholesterol, high blood pressure and stroke for the simple reason that, in our view, the evidence of efficacy just isn't there.

We've also examined many of the new non-conventional approaches to reversing heart disease, including the best diets, the best lifestyle changes and the importance of social connection for heart health. Instead of fad diets promising miracle cures or rigid dietary regimes that cut out virtually all fat, in the last third of this book we provide a practical Healthy Heart programme of diet, supplements, lifestyle changes and alternative treatments demonstrated to work, that the entire family can follow.

Although medicine considers that any adversary as formidable as heart disease can be defeated only by the most sophisticated of drugs, surgery and medical gadgetry, we hope this book will persuade that you that many far more gentle alternative treatments may actually be more effective in treating all manner of heart conditions.

Alternative medicine, which often employs a holistic approach, even tackles one under-appreciated cause of heart disease: social isolation. For all its clever technology, modern medicine doesn't take into account that many people with heart disease are literally dying of a broken heart.

May this book help you keep yours intact and in rude health for the whole of your life.

||||||||||||||||||||||||||||||||||||

Part I

THE MYTH OF PREVENTION

Chapter 1

THE MYTH ABOUT FATS AND CHOLESTEROL

A high cholesterol level is potentially dangerous and can lead to heart disease, or so doctors tell us. Cholesterol, we're told, usually comes from a high-fat diet. It's deposited within arteries, causing them to thicken and narrow. In turn, this will eventually block the blood supply to the heart, causing a heart attack or stroke.

Cholesterol is a waxy substance found in your blood and every cell in your body. It helps to produce vitamin D, cell membranes, hormones and even the bile that aids digestion (*see pages 11–12*). And in addition to the cholesterol your body itself manufactures, cholesterol comes from your diet – in meat, for example, because it's a vital substance for animals as well.

The entire basis of preventative medicine for heart disease has been driven by the medical theory that the two major causes of all heart disease are either high blood pressure (hypertension) or 'hyperlipidaemia', which is high levels of low-density lipoprotein (LDL) cholesterol (the so-called 'bad' cholesterol) caused by diabetes, smoking, poor diet, physical inactivity, obesity, drinking excessive amounts of alcohol and genetic factors.

Unfortunately, this universally accepted theory, which launched the multibillion-dollar statin and low-fat food industry, is poorly supported by the facts. Indeed, the facts support the very reverse of this idea.

Every year, Americans spend around $26 billion (£17 billion) on statin drugs and at least double that amount on low-fat foods, spreads and drinks (such as low-fat milk) to reduce levels of 'bad' artery-clogging LDL cholesterol. But on this front we've been the victims of medicine's biggest ever red herring, waging war for 50 years on a fat that can save our lives, keep us healthy and even protect us from the very heart disease it's supposed to cause.

Astonishingly, the theory that high-fat foods like meat and dairy can raise our cholesterol and so cause a build-up of fatty tissue in our arteries has never been proven. Yet it continues to be promulgated today – just as it has been since it was first mooted in the mid-1950s. As WebMD (www.webmd.com), one of the world's most popular medical websites, tells its visitors: 'LDL [low-density lipoprotein] cholesterol can't help being bad – it's just its chemical makeup. LDL cholesterol is an important part of the process of narrowing arteries. ... An LDL cholesterol-lowering diet is low in saturated fat and dietary cholesterol. Adding fibre and plant sterols, like cholesterol-lowering margarine, can further lower LDL levels.' The site disregards 40 years of research demonstrating that each of these statements is false. Two recent studies confirm what a minority of heart specialists have always suspected: high-fat foods don't raise levels of cholesterol.

In fact, researchers are now discovering something that contradicts the entire cholesterol theory: cholesterol actually protects against heart disease. And the 'bad' LDL type – as distinct from 'good' high-density lipoprotein (HDL) cholesterol, which mops up its apparently evil relation – has a special part to play in this.

Cholesterol sceptics

The first part of the hypothesis – that a high-fat diet causes heart disease – was recently discredited in a 10-year study of 3,630 middle-aged men and women in Costa Rica, who were split into 1,815 'cases' who had suffered a heart attack and the same number of healthy 'controls'.

Researchers at Brown University in Providence, Rhode Island, discovered that both groups consumed similar levels of dairy products like milk, cheese, yoghurt and butter, which are full of supposedly harmful saturated fats. Some in the healthy group were voracious consumers of high-fat dairy, eating up to 593g/day – yet none of them had suffered a heart attack. The researchers concluded that 'the evidence is not there' to support the high fats/heart disease theory.[1]

In an earlier study, researchers at Texas A&M University had gone a step further: they discovered that 'bad' LDL cholesterol is actually good for us. In a study of 52 adults aged 60 to 69 years who were in good health but not physically active, those with high levels of LDL cholesterol developed the most lean muscle mass after vigorously working out.

As team leader Steve Riechman said, 'The truth is, cholesterol is all good. You simply can't remove all the "bad" cholesterol from your body without serious problems occurring. People often say "I want to get rid of all my bad cholesterol," but the fact is, if you did so, you would die.'[2]

Although findings like these have been published in medical journals since the 1960s, invariably they've been dismissed as anomalous or just plain wrong because they don't fit within the prevailing cholesterol-is-bad-for-you paradigm.

A minority of researchers and doctors, including those who have joined groups like The International Network of Cholesterol Skeptics (THINCS), headed by Danish researcher Dr Uffe Ravnskov, has maintained for years that cholesterol is vital to our heart, our body and our mental health. If that's true, it's not surprising that statin drugs, which reduce our levels of cholesterol, have been cited as a cause of muscle damage, dementia, general cognitive decline and even life-threatening diseases such as cancer.

But, if the fatty foods-cholesterol-atherosclerosis theory is wrong, how did it ever see the light of day?

Back to the 1950s

By 1950, heart disease had become the major killer in the West. In the USA, it was responsible for a third of all deaths, mostly from heart attack. More than 500,000 Americans were dying every year from a heart attack compared with just 3,000 in 1930.

What had caused this sudden epidemic? After the deprivations of the Second World War, diet and nutrition were both large in the public mind, and researchers quickly latched on to the idea that the food we eat must somehow be responsible for heart disease. Some scientists suggested that the epidemic was caused by the rise of hydrogenated vegetable oils found in 'newer' foods like margarine and biscuits, and that heart disease would decline if we returned to the less processed foods, such as butter, that our grandparents ate.

But there was another food theory on the horizon. David Kritchevsky, a researcher at the Wistar Institute in Philadelphia, Pennsylvania, demonstrated that cholesterol fed to rabbits caused atherosclerosis.[3] Subsequently, he told the American Oil Chemists Society that polyunsaturated fats – found in vegetable and corn oils, soya beans, and safflower and sunflower seeds – could reduce cholesterol levels.

Within two years the 'lipid hypothesis' had gained momentum. The American Heart Association (AHA) launched the so-called 'Prudent Diet' in 1956 – in which corn oil, margarine, chicken and cold cereal replaced butter, lard, beef and eggs – in a nationwide TV broadcast across the USA. One of the experts on the show was Ancel Keys, a researcher at the University of Minnesota, whose name was to become synonymous with the cholesterol hypothesis.

In 1958, Keys launched the hugely influential Seven Countries Study, which gave birth to the idea of the 'Mediterranean diet' and gave further credence to the lipid theory. In surveys carried out between 1958 and 1970, he examined the fat intakes of seven countries, including the USA, Japan, Finland and the former Yugoslavia, and allegedly demonstrated a clear correlation between mortality due to heart disease and the percentage of calories from dietary fat.[4]

From this extraordinarily limited data came medicine's initial hypothesis that high dietary fat intakes cause high levels of cholesterol in the blood which, in turn, fur up arteries and set up a chain of events that eventually culminates in heart attack or stroke. According to this reasoning, heart attacks and strokes could largely be prevented by lowering blood cholesterol levels by either drugs or limiting fat intake.

But later analyses of the study by Ravnskov and others demonstrated that Keys had been highly selective in his data and had cherry-picked only what supported the high-fats hypothesis. In fact, he'd gathered data from 22 countries and ignored the results from 15 of them. If Keys had included all of the collected data, the diet-cholesterol link would have disappeared, says Ravnskov in his book *The Cholesterol Myths* (New Trends Publishing, Washington, DC, 2000) – a tome so reviled by the medical establishment that a copy was burned during a live TV show in Finland.

Keys took up an influential position on the advisory committee of the AHA, and his fats theory gained momentum. By 1984 it had been accepted as fact and a new healthy diet was born – and, with it, a new production line of low-fat foods and drinks.

No link with heart disease

Ravnskov wasn't the only one having difficulty finding a connection between high-fat foods and heart disease. To its embarrassment and cost, the US Surgeon General's Office had the same problem. For 11 years – from 1988 to 1999 – four project officers worked on a definitive report on fats and heart disease, assured that the science was there. Finally, the last project officer issued a letter announcing that the report would never be issued.

Bill Harlan, associate director of the Office of Disease Prevention (ODP) of the US National Institutes of Health (NIH), who helped oversee the project, said, 'The report was initiated with a preconceived opinion of the conclusions,' and admitted that the science behind those opinions was not supportive.[5]

But it's not only that a high-fat diet doesn't raise levels of cholesterol: the next part of the theory – that cholesterol causes heart disease and heart attack – also fails to stack up. Ravnskov has identified around 15 studies that clearly demonstrate that cholesterol plays no role in the development of heart disease.[6] Even the prestigious Framingham Heart Study, which has tracked the heart health of the population of this small town in Massachusetts since 1948, concluded that high cholesterol levels didn't predict fatal heart attacks. In fact, the researchers found quite the reverse: people with low cholesterol levels were more likely to die of heart disease.[7]

Nor could a connection be found in a study of 997 people aged 70 and older. High cholesterol levels weren't associated with any increased risk of death from any cause, including heart disease or heart attack, the researchers concluded.[8]

The high-cholesterol paradox

In fact, when examining the link between high cholesterol in the general population and the incidence of heart disease worldwide, researchers from the World Health Organization (WHO) discovered a giant paradox: countries with the highest levels of cholesterol had the lowest death rates from heart disease, while those with the lowest cholesterol levels had the highest death rates.

The biggest surprises were seen in the Aboriginals of Australia and in the Swiss. The Aboriginals have some of the world's lowest cholesterol levels – averaging 4.9mmol/L (88.2mg/dL) – yet they also have the highest death rates from heart disease, at around 1,100 deaths per 100,000 people per year. They confound all the other standard measures of heart risk too. Their blood pressure is a healthy 127/77mmHg and their average body mass index (BMI) is a lean 23.2kg/m^2 – both far 'healthier' than averages in the UK. And yet their mortality from heart disease is nearly four times greater than the UK's.

At the other end of the spectrum sits Switzerland. The Swiss have some of the highest cholesterol levels in the world, at around 6.4mmol/L (115.2mg/dL). This level wouldn't only trigger a statin prescription, it would probably also have every heart specialist scrambling to your side. Despite that, the Swiss enjoy some of the lowest rates of heart disease-related death, at just 150 per 100,000 people.

The statistics are as contrary as the science. The percentage of UK men with what are considered 'dangerous' levels of cholesterol – 5mmol/L (90mg/dL) or higher – has fallen from 75 per cent in 1994 to 58 per cent in 2008. The biggest drop has been in the 75-plus age range, with just 39 per cent of them having dangerously high levels compared with 79 per cent in 1994. Yet despite this dramatic decrease in the numbers of people with high cholesterol, the incidence of heart disease has remained stubbornly fixed over the 10 years up to 2008. In fact, the level of heart disease has risen slightly in the over-75s, the group with the most dramatic reductions in cholesterol, from 24 per cent in 1988 to around 30 per cent in 2008.

What is cholesterol?

Cholesterol is a fat, or lipid, carried in our blood, produced by the liver from saturated fat in our diet, some absorbed directly from cholesterol-rich foods like egg yolks and dairy products. It's an important 'building block' of life, a component of every single one of our cells. Cholesterol consists of LDL (low-density lipoprotein) cholesterol, VLDL (very low-density lipoprotein) cholesterol and HDL (high-density lipoprotein) cholesterol. Both LDL and VLDL are considered the real culprits behind heart disease, while HDL actually protects against heart disease by drawing cholesterol away from arterial walls and back to the liver.

Because it's carried in the blood, cholesterol is measured in millimoles per litre of blood (mmol/L); or milligrams per decilitre (mg/dL) in the US. No one in medicine really knows just what constitutes a dangerous level of blood cholesterol, but any level of cholesterol above 6mmol/L (108mg/dL) is considered high, although these days doctors on both sides of the Atlantic will write out a prescription for a cholesterol-lowering statin drug on any reading above 5–5.2mmol/L (90–93.6mg/dL). In truth, 'healthy' cholesterol levels vary according to the latest medical fashion. The average total cholesterol level in the UK is 6.1mmol/Ln (109.8mg/dL), while medicine currently believes that the 'optimal' total is 5mmol/L (90mg/dL). Of that quantity, HDL or 'good' cholesterol constitutes about 1.3mmol/L (23.4mg/dL), although the optimal level according to your doctor is anything above 2mmol/L (36mg/dL). A 'bad' LDL level is typically 3.5mmol/L (63mg/dL), although any reading above 4mmol/L (72mg/dL) will trigger a prescription for statin. Around 20 years ago in America a healthy total cholesterol level was considered no more than 7mmol/L (126mg/dL), but this fell to 6.5mmol/L (117mg/dL) around 10 years ago and today the drive is relentlessly downwards, with some experts calling for a new 'healthy' total cholesterol level of just 2.5mmol/L (45mg/dL). Researchers at the prestigious Harvard Medical School want to see the average LDL cholesterol level halved in the USA: '... perhaps someday,' they say, 'there will be a consensus that nearly everyone should make aggressive attempts to lower their LDL cholesterol with statins.'[9] But researchers at the University of Michigan argue that the current recommendations for LDL levels are entirely arbitrary and have no scientific validity.[10]

It remains unclear what role, if any, cholesterol in general – and the LDL variety in particular – plays in heart disease, although the conventional view is still that LDL cholesterol serves no useful purpose. As one US hospital website maintains, 'When too much LDL (bad) cholesterol circulates in the blood, it can slowly build up in the inner walls of the arteries that feed the heart and brain ... [and] can form plaque, a thick, hard deposit that can narrow the arteries ...'[11] The medical party line is that people get 'too much' LDL cholesterol when they eat fatty foods, among other things.

Cholesterol keeps us alive

All of our cells apart from neurons (nerve cells) contain cholesterol, which is synthesized by the liver. Both kinds of cholesterol are needed to:

⇨   Create brain synapses, which connect our nerve cells

⇨   Synthesize vitamin D from sunlight – for healthy bones and protection against various cancers

⇨ Keep our cells alive

⇨ Produce sex hormones

⇨ Make bile, which helps us digest our food.

Good guys and bad guys

Lipoproteins, the molecules that move cholesterol around the body, are often described as 'good' – the high-density lipoproteins (HDL) that remove cholesterol from cells and return it to the liver – and 'bad' – the low-density lipoproteins (LDL) that transport cholesterol from the liver to the cells. This suggests that when you have too little HDL and too much LDL, cholesterol isn't getting back to the liver, so it starts to collect in arteries.

Then there are triglycerides, a type of fat found in the bloodstream. Again, too much of this fat can cause narrowing of the arteries because of the build-up of fatty plaques in the artery walls, which eventually turns into a hardening of the arteries.

A healthy cholesterol profile supposedly consists of a high level of HDL and low levels of LDL and triglyceride. A relatively normal LDL level is considered 5.6–7.2mmol/L in the UK (100.8–129.6mg/dL in the USA) and a dangerous level is anything above 10.5mmol/L (189mg/dL). Similarly, a dangerous level of triglyceride is anything over 27.8mmol/L (500.4mg/dL), and a poor HDL level is one below 2.2mmol/L (39.6mg/dL).

The trouble is, real life doesn't fit with any of this. Researchers from the University of California at Los Angeles were astonished when they reviewed the cholesterol profiles of 136,905 patients admitted to hospital after a heart attack. Only a small minority had cholesterol levels in the danger range – in fact, most had ideal levels – yet all had suffered a heart attack.[12] Overall, 75 per cent of patients had healthy cholesterol levels, while their 'bad' LDL levels were well within the acceptable range and nearly half had levels of 'good' HDL cholesterol higher than 2.2mmol/L (39.6mg/dL).

In fact, such a failure of proof has been repeatedly found by other researchers through the years. One review of seven clinical studies and 16 observational studies, involving hundreds of thousands of people, failed to establish any meaningful association between cholesterol and heart disease.[13] Nor could Dutch researcher Robert Hoenselaar uncover any data to support the recommendations that cholesterol levels can be lowered by consuming a diet low in saturated fats.[14] What's more, after analyzing 76 studies of heart health and diet, involving close to 650,000 participants, researchers from Cambridge University in the UK could find absolutely no evidence to support the idea that the amount of saturated fat we eat has any impact on heart health.[15]

Inflammation overload

If fatty foods aren't the cause of our clogged arteries, then what is? Medicine has begun to accept that inflammation may be a cause of heart disease. Even conservative groups like the American Heart Association are recognizing the role of inflammation in heart disease, and studies have demonstrated clear associations. In one study comparing 506 men who had suffered a heart attack with 1,025 healthy controls, inflammation was a significant indicator of heart disease. Men with the highest levels of C-reactive protein

(CRP) in their blood – a recognized marker of inflammation – were more than twice as likely to have heart disease.[16]

Still, inflammation is not a cause: it's simply the body's immune response to stress and infection. In medicine, the concept of stress refers to any 'insult' to the body, such as a poor diet of processed foods, exposure to environmental pollutants or emotional stress due to tension, depression or feelings of isolation or helplessness (see Chapter 12).

What is inflammation?

The first reaction of doctors is to reduce inflammation, usually with anti-inflammatory drugs such as aspirin. It's the standard treatment taught at medical school – yet it's hopelessly out of step with the body and its natural healing mechanisms.

Inflammation is a good thing. It's the immune system's attempt to heal wounds and injuries, beat infection and protect joints from chronic diseases like arthritis. In an inflammatory response, plasma proteins and phagocytes (white blood cells) initiate tissue repair in the injured area. They also increase the rate of muscle regeneration.

Many chronic diseases are now being recognized as inflammatory or having an inflammatory element, including heart disease and even cancer. LDL or 'bad' cholesterol has a role to play in the inflammatory process in cardiovascular disease, when the heart and major arteries of the body may be damaged. In effect, LDL cholesterol is trying to repair damage to arterial walls, but ends up closing them by laying down plaque in an attempt to salvage them.

Cholesterol, the good guy

In fact, a new school of thought believes that LDL cholesterol plays a positive role in our health and wellbeing. As a marker of inflammation or infection-fighter, it's trying to repair damaged arteries – but ends up like the good guy trying to help out at the scene of the crime when the police barge in and accuse the wrong man.

If this idea is correct, then LDL cholesterol forms in our arteries to repair inflammatory damage caused by infection or stress – not by eating too much fatty food.

The importance of cholesterol has been borne out in a variety of studies showing no connection between levels of cholesterol and heart disease. For example, in a review of 19 studies from the USA, Europe, Israel and Japan, which included 68,406 deaths, many due to non-cardiovascular causes, all the victims had low levels of total cholesterol.[17] In another study, the chances of survival in patients with chronic heart failure were definitely related to their levels of cholesterol, but it was those with high levels who were far more likely to be alive than those with low levels.[18]

The health-keeping role of cholesterol becomes even more important as we get older. In a study of 724 participants with an average age of 89, each 1mmol/L (18mg/dL) increase in total cholesterol corresponded to a 15 per cent drop in the mortality rate. In other words, those who had the highest cholesterol levels lived the longest. Overall, cholesterol appeared to have a protective effect against cancer and infection.[19]

Cholesterol also helps us stay mentally sharp with age, protecting against dementia and cognitive decline. One study of 1,051 people aged 65 and older discovered that those suffering from dementia had significantly lower total, LDL and HDL cholesterol levels.[20]

In fact, your body needs so much cholesterol that the liver produces between four to five times the amount of cholesterol you get from food. In a biological process known as 'downregulation', the liver produces less cholesterol if your diet is high in fatty foods. Illustrating the importance of cholesterol, a victim of Smith-Lemli-Opitz syndrome (SLOS), a rare developmental disorder that causes very low cholesterol levels, can suffer from spontaneous abortion, multi-organ system failure and immediate death, congenital heart disease, frequent vomiting, blindness or visual impairment, deafness, pneumonia, or heart or liver failure leading to death.

Fluctuating cholesterol levels

Heart specialist Stephen Sinatra, assistant clinical professor of medicine at the University of Connecticut School of Medicine, began to question the cholesterol hypothesis when some of his patients with low cholesterol levels – some at just 7.2mmol/L (129.6mg/dL) – still went on to develop heart problems. Discussing this with his colleagues, he discovered that other cardiologists had noticed the same phenomenon. On researching the issue further, Sinatra discovered that:

⇨ The body makes cholesterol as needed, so when you eat more, the body makes less

⇨ Your cholesterol levels rise and fall throughout the day

⇨ Cholesterol levels rise in winter and drop in summer

⇨ Cholesterol rises following surgery, following an infection, when you're feeling stressed, and both during and after a heart attack.

'One reason for these variables,' says Sinatra, 'is that cholesterol serves as a healing agent. The body produces cholesterol when there is a healing job to do.'[21] This explains why cholesterol levels are high when people have heart problems or after they've suffered a heart attack. And as it's often found at the scene, it's been wrongly identified as the perpetrator.

Cholesterol isn't only a healing agent. As we age, it also appears to play an important role in longevity. A Dutch study found that people aged 85 and older with high cholesterol lived longer, and were also less likely to die of cancer or infection.[22] Sinatra believes that cholesterol only becomes a potential danger to arterial and heart health when it reaches levels as high as 17.8mmol/L (320.4mg/dL), nearly a third higher than the current levels at which US doctors prescribe statins. His view is supported by the Copenhagen City Heart Study, which looked at the health records of 19,698 residents from 1976 to 1988. Of these, 693 had suffered a heart attack within a five-year period, but cholesterol was directly linked to these heart attacks only when levels were so high that they were in the top 5 per cent recorded for all participants.[23] So, while it plays a part in heart problems, cholesterol's role may not be anywhere near as significant as the current medical thinking would have it.

Healthy high cholesterol

In the 1970s Dr George Mann of Vanderbilt University in Nashville, Tennessee, studied the diet and health of the Masai tribe in East Africa. Their diet was almost entirely made up of meat, blood and milk from their cattle – and yet their cholesterol levels were low and heart disease was almost unheard of.

Mann concluded that the cholesterol-heart disease theory was 'the greatest scam in the history of medicine'.[24] What he meant was that the food industry – and later the drugs industry – made a fortune from the theory. It continues to do so.

As well as a scam, it's also a tragedy. By attacking LDL cholesterol, we deplete the body's stores of a vital fat that's one of our biggest allies in the fight against inflammation and infection. It's especially needed as we get old, when it protects us against dementia and cognitive (mental) decline. Despite this, the elderly are especially targeted for cholesterol-lowering statins – as indeed they are for many drugs out there.

Dementia may be not only a symptom of old age, but the legacy of the greatest scam in the history of medicine.

|||||||||||||||||||||||||||||||||||||||||||

Chapter 2

THE MYTH OF DANGEROUS BLOOD PRESSURE LEVELS

Do you have high blood pressure (hypertension) that has the doctor reaching for the prescription pad? If so, you – like the millions of people taking powerful drugs to treat high and 'abnormal' blood pressure and prevent heart disease – are victims of another of medicine's great blunders in preventative medicine. Although high blood pressure is seen as one of the most common health risks we face as we grow older, the standard method of measuring it is so seriously flawed that many millions of people believe their health is in jeopardy when it isn't, and so are willingly taking drugs they don't need. Despite what doctors tell them, their health may not be at risk and they may have every chance of living just as long as people who have 'normal' blood pressure.

To make matters worse, there's no agreement in medicine about what a dangerous reading is, and it just got more complicated with the USA moving the goalposts again in 2014. This time, though – and for the first time ever – they have relaxed the criteria for starting drug therapy.

That said, the antihypertensive drugs given to patients with high blood pressure are still increasing their chances of suffering the very heart attack they believe the drugs are helping them to avoid. In fact, as we'll see in Chapter 7, one type of antihypertensive drug – calcium-channel blockers (CCBs) – actually trebles the risk.

Up and down with the times

Blood pressure is the force with which blood pushes against the walls of arteries. What's characterized as a 'healthy' blood pressure level varies according to the patient's age.

High blood pressure may be a precursor of heart attack, heart failure, stroke and kidney disease, according to modern medicine. We're told that around one in three adults has hypertension, often described by medicine as a 'silent killer'. Because there are no symptoms, blood pressure readings are the most common – and frequent – tests performed in medicine, often using a portable device called a 'sphygmomanometer', which includes a cuff wrapped around the patient's upper arm.

The standard cuff is a bladder in a cloth sleeve. Air is pumped into the bladder, either manually or through a self-measuring machine, until its pressure is higher than the pressure in your arm's main artery, so that it stops the flow of blood. When the air is released from the cuff's bladder, blood surges back into the artery. A medical assistant listens to this process through a stethoscope placed over your arm's main artery.

Blood pressure levels are determined by two readings made in millimetres of mercury (mmHg): systolic blood pressure measures arterial pressure when the heart beats; and diastolic blood pressure measures the pressure between heartbeats (at rest). These days a 'healthy' or 'normal' blood pressure reading is around 120/80mmHg (systolic blood pressure is the first number). If the systolic or diastolic reading or both are higher than this, the diagnosis is hypertension. The units 'mmHg' stand for 'millimetres of mercury'.

However, so-called normal or healthy blood pressure seems to change with the times. In the past, doctors gauged a healthy systolic blood pressure level as 100mmHg plus the age of the patient, so an acceptable reading for a 60-year-old was 160mmHg. The goalposts were then moved in 2003 as part of the current and more exacting definition of hypertension. At the same time, the US National Institutes of Health (NIH) also set a 'prehypertensive state' – which can be treated by lifestyle and dietary changes – at anything from 120/80 to 139/89mmHg, and drug therapy would begin with any reading from 140/90 to 159/99mmHg. Before 2003, a normal blood pressure was 128/80mmHg.

At the time, the lower normal blood pressure levels were not universally welcomed. As Dr Paul J. Rosch, former clinical professor of medicine at New York Medical College, said, 'All that these new guidelines essentially accomplish is to convert 45 million healthy Americans into new patients.'

The new lower threshold was good news, however, for the manufacturers of antihypertensive drugs like ACE (angiotensin-converting enzyme) inhibitors, calcium-channel blockers and diuretics ('water tablets'). Now, antihypertensive agents worth more than $26 billion (£17 billion) are prescribed every year throughout the developed world, making it one of the most successful drug groups prescribed today.

Up to December 2014 a dangerous high blood pressure reading was 140/90mmHg – but at that time the level was redefined as 150/90mmHg or higher in the USA for everyone aged 60 or over, the age group taking the majority of antihypertensive agents.[1]

In the UK a high blood pressure reading is still set at 140/90mmHg, although it too may follow the USA's more relaxed definition soon.

Raising the bar means that fewer people will be taking betablockers, antihypertensive agents that can themselves be killers. In a review and analysis of nine trials involving 10,529 patients taking betablockers before heart surgery – as recommended by both the American and European guidelines – the reviewers found a 27 per cent increase in deaths due to stroke and hypotension (dangerously low blood pressure) in patients who took these drugs.[2]

Fluctuating levels

Your blood pressure normally rises and falls throughout the day. It's highest in the morning, and it can also differ from one arm to the other. And your systolic reading – the first number – can rise by as much as 30mmHg just because you're waiting anxiously for the doctor to take a reading. In fact, this happens so frequently that the phenomenon has a name: 'white-coat hypertension'. Doctors are supposed to take this into account when they assess whether or not you need to start a course of antihypertensive drugs, but a good deal depends on the doctor and how much he or she toes the line.

How to take your own blood pressure

If you're worried about getting a false reading – and so starting drugs you don't actually need – you can monitor your own blood pressure by regularly checking it throughout the day at home. The best devices are the fully automatic digital monitors that measure your blood pressure at the upper arm rather than wrist or finger. Be sure to measure your upper arm circumference carefully and order the right size of cuff for your arm. Companies like Microlife, A&D Instruments, Boots, Braun, Citizen, Health & Life, Honsun (Suresign), Kinetik, Lloyds Pharmacy, Omron and Panasonic all make monitors that have been clinically approved.

The importance of systolic blood pressure

One important reason why the majority of prescriptions for hypertension are unnecessary is that doctors are prescribing them based on the wrong readings. Systolic pressure is the only figure that matters in the over-50s, according to one theory, called isolated systolic hypertension (ISH), while the diastolic level is all but irrelevant as we get older, and this is especially true for men.

According to the prestigious Framingham Heart Study, an ongoing study started in 1948 of cardiovascular disease in more than 5,000 people living in the small town of Framingham, Massachusetts, an estimated 65 per cent of all hypertension cases in the elderly are caused by raised systolic pressure together with an increase in pulse pressure (the difference between the systolic and diastolic pressures), although the need to focus solely on the systolic measurement has not been translated into clinical practice.[3]

Researchers from the University of Minneapolis estimate that 100 million Americans – and by their reckoning, around 20 million Brits as well – have what's considered an 'abnormal' blood pressure reading that poses no threat to either health or longevity, but still places them in a category for an antihypertensive drug.

In uncovering one of medicine's biggest mistakes, the researchers – led by Brent Taylor – studied the health and longevity of nearly 14,000 Americans aged 25 to 75 with different blood pressure levels, and analyzed their systolic and diastolic levels by age and mortality rate.[4]

They found a complex picture. Among the over-50s there was a direct and step-wise link between diastolic blood pressure and death. As the diastolic pressure increased, so did the risk of death, especially with readings higher than 90mmHg – but the risk disappeared completely when the systolic reading was factored in. Having a normal systolic reading neutralized a diastolic level that conventional medicine considered life-threatening.

In fact, the researchers found that systolic pressure was a far more important gauge of health risk among the over-50s, whereas the diastolic pressure meant nothing. The reverse was true for the under-50s. This suggests a completely new way of assessing blood pressure, one that is dependent on age and perhaps gender, as the systolic reading seems even more significant in men.

Systolic pressure and ageing

The importance of the ISH theory has been growing over recent years as researchers discover how accurate a predictor it is, especially for older patients. A team at the University of Leuven in Belgium concluded that doctors were misjudging the health dangers – and prescribing antihypertensives inappropriately – when they looked at both systolic and diastolic blood pressure.

In a review of eight separate studies, the Belgian researchers examined the health records of nearly 16,000 people aged 60 years and older with blood pressure readings of 160/95mmHg or higher. They found that only the systolic reading was an accurate predictor of fatal and non-fatal heart complications. Every 10mmHg increase in systolic pressure correlated with a nearly 10 per cent increase in heart risk while, yet again, the diastolic reading provided no helpful indication of future heart health problems.[5]

Japanese researchers had similar findings indicating that systolic pressure alone was an accurate indicator of heart problems in both the young and old. A 19-year study involving nearly 3,800 men of all ages revealed that raised systolic pressure was an independent risk factor for cardiovascular disease, whereas a raised diastolic reading was insignificant, no matter what the age. A high systolic pressure increased the risk of cardiovascular disease by 1.5 times in the 30-to-64-year-olds, by 1.7 times in the 64-to-74-year-olds and by 1.2 times in those aged over 75.[6]

A French study went further and suggested that a 'normal' diastolic reading could be more dangerous than a higher one. In a review of nearly 125,000 men and women – all of whom were healthy at the beginning of the eight-year study – the researchers found a direct correlation between an increase in systolic readings and heart disease and death. And the diastolic measure was irrelevant if the systolic reading was normal. Even a high diastolic reading –

normally considered a sign of hypertension – was found to have no bearing on future health.

In fact, a normal diastolic reading was more dangerous in men (but not in women) who had raised systolic levels compared with having a mild-to-moderate increase in diastolic pressure.[7]

Inaccurate readings

A failure to understand the significance of systolic pressure is only part of the problem, since doctors, as already suggested, often don't get an accurate reading to begin with. This may be down to several factors – from faulty equipment to time of day and what the patient was doing before being measured.

One US study that tracked the progress of patients in a hospital emergency room found that blood pressure readings were wrong in almost every case. Exploring further, the researchers discovered that the automated blood-pressure-measuring equipment was faulty and failed to meet even the most basic criteria laid down by the international Association for the Advancement of Medical Instrumentation (AAMI).[8]

In another study of men aged over 65, most were victims of 'pseudohypertension', an incorrect or faulty reading of a high blood pressure due to arterial stiffness (or, in medical-speak, a lack of 'arterial compliance') often seen in older adults, or some other error. While the BP cuff was reading a level of 180/100mmHg, the true level – on average – was just 165/85mmHg, which some doctors still consider normal in such elderly patients.[9]

Even when the equipment isn't faulty, it can be hopelessly inaccurate. Professor William White of the University of Connecticut's Pat and Jim Calhoun Cardiology Center, who specializes in clinical hypertension and vascular diseases, has described the sphygmomanometer as 'medicine's crudest investigation'.

As he points out, blood pressure can vary by as much as 30mmHg over the course of a day.[10] It can increase with physical exertion, stress of any kind – including the stress of 'white-coat hypertension' – because of the room temperature, a full bladder, or eating, drinking or smoking within an hour of having the test. Even an animated conversation can temporarily raise your blood pressure by as much as 50 per cent.

People who have their test in the morning are likely to register far higher levels than when the test is carried out in the afternoon, and some patients are encouraged to wear a blood pressure monitor for 24 hours to get the most accurate reading. A night-time read-out of such a day-long test is the one that will give the most accurate readings of all. In one study of people who performed such 'ambulatory monitoring' (at home or out of hospital), the night-time readings proved to be the best for predicting health problems.[11]

Your blood pressure can even vary between arms. The most accurate readings are taken from the left arm, and researchers have found a difference of as much as 5mmHg between the left- and right-arm readings in the same patient. In one report, the biggest difference noted between the two arms was 20mmHg.[12]

The final analysis

For a condition that affects so many of us, medicine's understanding of hypertension is lamentable. To summarize, conventional medicine:

⇨ Fails to understand the significance of the systolic/diastolic balance as we age

⇨ Often misreads blood pressure levels

⇨ Sets the threshold for hypertension at too low a level

⇨ Doesn't appreciate that higher blood pressures can be a normal part of the ageing process.

Despite these shortcomings, the American Heart Association says that hypertension is 'easily detected and usually controllable' while at the same time admitting that the death rate from hypertension rose by 19.5 per cent between 1996 and 2006 in the USA.

Because it has no real answers in its battle against hypertension, medicine is behaving like a policeman in a banana republic: it's too forceful, intrusive, interfering and aggressive. A more conservative and thoughtful approach might serve both doctors and patients far better.

High blood pressure is a symptom of our modern way of life. Processed foods and a sedentary lifestyle can all add up to an unhealthy blood pressure reading. As you'll see, there are plenty of other ways to modify your diet and lifestyle gently that are far safer, and work considerably better, than swallowing a pill.

||||||||||||||||||||||||||||||||||||||||||||||

Chapter 3

ASPIRIN TO PREVENT STROKE: SPIN, NOT SCIENCE

Often without warning, life can be torn apart by the sudden trauma to the brain caused by a stroke. The third biggest killer in the West, stroke is the most important cause of adult disability.[1] Among those aged over 65, it's the second most common cause of death after heart disease and, as it's essentially a 'heart attack' in the brain caused by a problem involving blood circulation, it's often lumped together with heart disease. And as with atherosclerosis and high blood pressure, medicine purports to have successful preventative medicine for it – a claim based far more on spin than real science.

Stroke is a non-specific, collective term for symptoms like paralysis, perceptual loss, speech difficulties and visual problems that are the result of damage to brain tissue caused by one of three situations.

Most commonly, a blood clot gradually builds up in a brain artery (arterial occlusion), eventually blocking the blood supply to the related part of the brain (this blockage is called infarction). By starving this area of oxygen, a cerebral thrombosis, or blood clot, leaves its victim with a variable degree of tissue damage, or frequently death. But this may also be the result of atherosclerosis, or narrowing of the arteries. Often, both atherosclerosis and arterial occlusion are acting together, as the formation of blood clots in the brain can be the result of platelets forming in response to damaged tissue in the lining of blood vessels. In the West, 85 per cent of strokes are the result of blood clots.[2] Blockages in the brain may also be due to a clot that has originated elsewhere in the body – usually in the heart or deep veins in the legs – and travelled upwards, causing what's known in medical-speak as a cerebral embolism.

A cerebral haemorrhage can cause a stroke because, when a blood vessel in the brain ruptures, the bleeding damages the associated area of the brain. High blood pressure can lead to such haemorrhage, usually through an aneurysm – local 'ballooning' of an artery, which causes it to burst. The extreme force of the blood spurting from an artery can damage the delicate brain tissue as well as compress and impair the adjacent areas. The degree of disability and loss of basic physical and mental skills after a stroke depends largely on the duration and site of the trauma.

No disorder is more confounding to medical science, because stroke can't be pinned down to one single treatable cause. Instead, it's influenced by a number of different factors that may be both organic (the physical state of the body) and iatrogenic (caused by medical examination or treatment). As a result, stroke prevention often takes a rather haphazard course and, in spite of the vast amounts of money that have been poured into the study of stroke and related vascular disorders, there's still very little known about this devastating disorder.[3]

Aspirin to prevent stroke

Even people who think twice about taking a pharmaceutical don't give a moment's thought to popping an aspirin every morning. After all, it's the ultimate 'just-in-case' lifestyle pill, supposedly offering protection against heart disease, especially stroke, and doctors regularly recommend it as part of a general health regime to all their patients who are 50-plus, as a big part of preventative medicine against heart disease. Long gone are the days when it was primarily reached for as a painkiller. It's probably also the most popular preventative medicine of modern times, with around 100 billion pills swallowed every year around the world to prevent heart disease and stroke. The elderly are especially encouraged to take aspirin to prevent cardiovascular problems such as heart failure and stroke, and it's even been touted as a way to prevent colorectal (bowel) cancer.

But major new research shows that the risks and benefits of routine aspirin use make for a very worrying picture: it could be costing as many lives as it saves.

Stroke fatalities in the UK have fallen over the past 20 years, and aspirin has been championed as one of the significant factors in the decline. But the figures have excluded deaths among the over-75s – and these have quadrupled over the same period. Professor Peter Rothwell, of the Stroke Prevention Research Unit at Oxford University, published a study in 2007 suggesting that aspirin could be one of the major causes of stroke in the over-75 age group.

Overall, Rothwell discovered a sevenfold increase in intracerebral haemorrhagic stroke (bleeding in the brain) in that age group, and this coincided with a massive increase in the use of a non-steroidal anti-inflammatory drug (NSAID), such as aspirin, to help thin the blood. Between 1981 and 1984 just 4 per cent of healthy people were taking the drug as a just-in-case measure, whereas between 2002 and 2006 this had risen dramatically to 40 per cent of the population.

Rothwell believes this is more than coincidence. As he states, 'There are elderly people who take aspirin as a lifestyle choice, and, in that situation, the trials have shown there's no benefit. And what our study suggests is that, particularly in the very elderly, the risks of aspirin outweigh the benefits.'[4]

'We have found that there is a fine balance between benefits and risks from regular aspirin use in primary prevention of cardiovascular disease,' points out Professor Aileen Clarke, who headed a team of investigators at Warwick Medical School in Coventry, UK.[5] Although the benefits of taking aspirin are certainly real, they're possibly far less impressive than doctors would have us believe. Taking a daily aspirin can reduce the rate of major cardiovascular events like heart attacks by around 10 per cent, and coronary heart disease by 15 per cent, the Warwick researchers calculated. That translates to 33 to 46 fewer deaths for every 100,000 people who take an aspirin every day for 10 years.

The real problem is that aspirin giveth – but it taketh away just as readily. On assessing 27 randomized controlled trials, the Warwick team also found that the drug increases the rate of gastrointestinal (GI) bleeding by 37 per cent and the risk of haemorrhagic stroke by 38 per cent. Convert that into numbers, and it means there are 117 extra cases of GI bleeding per 100,000 patient-years of taking aspirin and up to 10 additional cases of stroke, which is debilitating at best and fatal at worst. (A patient-year is calculated from the number of study patients multiplied by the number of years of the study, divided by the number of events being studied.)

GI blues

Most patients taking just-in-case aspirin (or some other NSAID) know it may cause GI bleeding, but few realize the seriousness of the effect or that it can be fatal. In fact, aspirin is seen as such a 'safe' drug that users don't associate it with their GI bleeds.

Researchers from the Eastern Virginia Medical School estimate that the drug is killing 20,000 Americans every year from GI complications – yet none is being recorded as an aspirin-related death. They base this estimate on a series of interviews conducted at a hospital specializing in GI problems. Only about one in five patients taking aspirin had reported the fact to the hospital, because they didn't consider it important enough to mention.

'This reflects a common misperception that these medications are insignificant or benign when actually their chronic use, particularly among the elderly and those with conditions such as arthritis, is linked to serious and potentially fatal GI injury and bleeding,' said Dr David Johnson, one of the researchers.[6]

Extrapolating those figures worldwide, aspirin could be responsible for 100,000 deaths and 500,000 emergency hospital treatments each year – and yet it's not being blamed for any of them. This is a far cry from the official figures estimating that NSAIDs, including aspirin, ibuprofen and naproxen, are responsible for around 7,600 deaths a year.[7]

While any death is one too many, in medical-speak the casualty rate is 'acceptable' because of the many more lives NSAIDs supposedly save each year from premature death due to heart attack, stroke and – now – cancer. In fact, the American Heart Association reckons that aspirin is saving the lives of up to 10,000 people who would otherwise be among the 900,000 casualties lost each year in the USA alone due to heart disease. The Association points to research suggesting that aspirin prolongs the lives of people who have already suffered a heart attack or stroke, or those who run the risk of recurring blockages in their arteries.

But the scales tip the other way when the true numbers of deaths and emergency treatments are factored in. As America's Food and Drug Administration (FDA) spokesperson Debra Bowen put it, 'Physicians really need to look at aspirin in the context of complete care, as part of a whole treatment plan for people at risk of heart attack or stroke.'

And Dr Peter Coleman of the UK's Stroke Association agrees: 'If you are healthy and have a low risk of heart disease or stroke, the increased risk from side-effects of aspirin is likely to outweigh the benefits of preventing stroke.'

This throws into question its casual use as a prophylactic, a just-in-case remedy, and it's difficult to see just who benefits from this practice. If the healthy shouldn't be taking aspirin, then it's already being taken inappropriately 40 per cent of the time. The under-65s run the risk of GI harm for a benefit that seems dubious and unproven, while the over-75s – the group believed to gain the most from its regular use – are more likely to suffer a fatal stroke.

The story of aspirin

Aspirin holds an unusual place in trademark law. As 'Aspirin' with a capital 'A', it's a protected brand name owned by Bayer, the German pharmaceutical giant. As 'aspirin', it's a generic drug that can be used in countries where Aspirin is not trademark-protected. Around 50 other over-the-counter preparations contain aspirin, using either that name or 'ASA', which stands for 'acetylsalicylic acid', Aspirin's generic name.

Aspirin was the very first drug in the NSAID family when Bayer began marketing it in 1899, along with another of the company's discoveries: heroin. Its principal ingredient is salicylic acid, derived from willow tree bark and the herb meadowsweet. Willow tree bark was also recognized by Hippocrates as a pain-reliever and antipyretic (fever-reducer) as long ago as the 5th century BC.

Chemists at Bayer were successful in synthesizing salicylic acid with the common chemical acetic anhydride, so giving Aspirin its generic name.

Despite its widespread use and popularity, no one understood how the drug worked until 1971, when John Vane (1927–2004), a British pharmacologist then working at the Wellcome Research Laboratories in southeast London, had his prize-winning insight. Vane had the flash of inspiration that aspirin might suppress the production of prostaglandins and thromboxanes – hormone-like lipids involved in many physiological functions. For this work he went on to share the Nobel Prize for Medicine in 1982.

Today we globally consume around 35,000 tons of aspirin every year, amounting to around 100 billion tablets – a figure that's increasing each year by 15 per cent.

Aspirin continues to be viewed as a benign painkiller, which has helped promote its growing use at a time when bad news and scares have hounded other NSAIDs and COX-2 inhibitors, a newer type of painkiller. The COX-2 painkiller Vioxx was withdrawn from the market after it was found to cause heart problems – some fatal. It was the subject of the largest civil lawsuit in history until its manufacturer Merck settled with a $4.85 billion (£3.1 billion) payout to around 50,000 families who had lost a family member to the drug.

Aspirin in the balance

Aspirin has been dogged by its own fair share of side-effects. The most common are stomach bleeding and other GI problems, but also stroke, anaemia, ulcers, liver damage, hives, wheezing, tinnitus (ringing in the ears), chronic catarrh, headache, confusion, and hypotension (abnormally low blood pressure) followed by collapse. Asthmatics have also died from a severe attack after taking aspirin.

And the real picture could be even grimmer. Given that so many deaths and injuries haven't been officially attributed to aspirin, it may be that the risks/rewards balance is in reality biased more heavily towards risks, outweighing the benefits.

||||||||||||||||||||||||||||||||||||||||||||

Chapter 4

THE UNHEALTHY PLATE

Most attempts at preventative medicine for heart attack, high blood pressure and stroke fail for one simple reason: the dietary advice that Westerners are given by their governments and by the medical community is neither good for your heart nor, indeed, for the rest of you.

Concerned by the epidemics of heart disease and other degenerative conditions, departments within the US and UK governments came up with the idea of using an image of a plate divided up like slices of a pie to show the different types and ideal proportions of foods we should be eating for optimal health. The plan on both sides of the Atlantic was to let the picture say a thousand words.

The UK's 'eatwell plate' is the more detailed of the two, using specific examples from each of the different food groups (eggs, fish and meat on the protein side of the plate, for example).

According to the UK eatwell plate, our diet should be roughly:

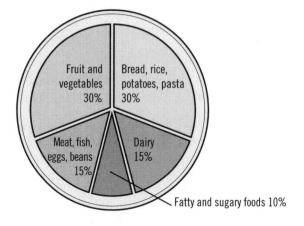

The UK eatwell plate

⇨ 15 per cent protein (eggs, meat, fish, beans and other protein alternatives)

⇨ 15 per cent dairy and milk

⇨ 30 per cent fruit and vegetables

⇨ 30 per cent grains (bread and other cereals), pasta and potatoes

⇨ 10 per cent foods high in fat and sugar.

MyPlate, the US version, shows a plate simply divided into five food groups, presented as four differently sized and coloured slices – indicating fruits, vegetables, grains and protein – with a glass on the side to represent dairy.

As First Lady Michelle Obama remarked on unveiling MyPlate in 2011, 'Parents don't have the time to measure out exactly three ounces of chicken or look up how much rice or broccoli is in a serving ... But we do have time to take a look at our kids' plates.'

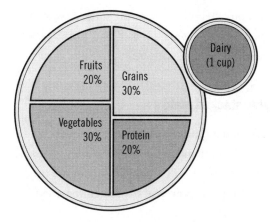

The US MyPlate

In the USA, the coloured sections are broadly meant to represent:

⇨ 30 per cent grains

⇨ 30 per cent vegetables

⇨ 20 per cent fruit

⇨ 20 per cent protein

⇨ 1 cup of dairy (including milk, yoghurt and cheese).

Flawed science

Both the US MyPlate and British eatwell plate are based on the long-standing received wisdom that fat makes you fat and carbohydrates are a comparatively benign alternative source of energy.[1]

But the low-fat advocates have overlooked one other essential ingredient: the role of refined carbohydrates and sugar in weight gain. As unbelievable as it seems to us now, they simply assumed that these components of diet had nothing to do with being overweight or indeed with heart disease.

A highly stacked plate

The recommendations of the eatwell plate and MyPlate both betray the heavy hand of the food-industry giants. There's no doubt that the high levels of carbohydrates are the result of commercial pressure from the powerful manufactured-food industry.

In assembling earlier versions of its food icon, the US government found it unnecessary to deny that the public relations agency (Porter Novelli) it hired to help create the icon also counted food manufacturers among its clients. And the bulk of manufactured food relies on refined carbohydrates, which are allowed on both plates.

Another commercial pressure was undoubtedly from the dairy industry. The eatwell plate calls for up to 15 per cent of dairy a day, clearly ignoring the copious research linking pasteurized and homogenized dairy products to allergies and even a greater risk of cancer, especially ovarian and prostate cancers.[2]

Although the ostensible reason for the inclusion of dairy was the prevention of osteoporosis (brittle bones), the evidence for that is so far inconclusive. One comprehensive study in Boston, Massachusetts, following nearly 80,000 women aged 34–59 for 12 years found that high intakes of dairy failed to protect against bone fractures.[3]

Harvard disagrees

When an earlier version of MyPlate, devised as a food pyramid, was released, Meir J. Stampfer, chairman of the Department of Epidemiology at Harvard's School of Public Health, and Walter C. Willett, a Harvard professor of nutrition, complained that it didn't pass scientific muster. What follows are all the things they described as wrong with the US version of a healthy plate, which equally apply to the UK's eatwell plate.

Mistake 1: The recommendations are based on the persistent and flawed notion that dietary fat of any sort leads to heart disease

Stampfer and Willett concluded that the scientific evidence fails to show a strong link between fat intake/cholesterol and heart disease or stroke. Healthy fats, whether monounsaturated or polyunsaturated, actually lower the risk of heart disease, Stampfer contends – and indeed, according to the latest evidence, saturated fats do not clog the arteries as we have long been led to believe.[4] The well-known ongoing Framingham Heart Study, which has followed a small-town population in Massachusetts for decades, revealed that the more saturated fat, cholesterol and calories consumed, the lower the blood cholesterol.[5]

Mistake 2: The two plates don't acknowledge the importance of saturated fats in the diet

According to Weston A. Price Foundation's Sally Fallon and the late fats expert Dr Mary Enig, saturated fats perform critical functions in the body, such as protecting bony surfaces, cushioning internal organs, strengthening cell membranes, building and protecting the nervous system, brain and liver, and helping to protect against osteoporosis – to name but a few. Saturated fats may also suppress tumour formation.[6] Placing unnecessary limits on consumption of fats can lead to gallstones and many other health problems. Restriction of saturated fat in particular has been identified as a cause of fatigue, poor concentration, depression and even weight gain, because the serotonin receptors in the brain need cholesterol to function properly.[7] Studies of a variety of native populations have rates of saturated fat consumption greater by several orders of magnitude than what's currently recommended, yet they still have far lower rates of heart disease (*see page 48*).

Mistake 3: The plates offer no information on levels of vital essential fatty acids, which tend to form too small a percentage of the average British and American processed diet

All fats receive a bad press, despite ample research indicating the substantial health benefits derived from natural fats like omega-3 essential fatty acids (EFAs).[8] These fatty acids, stored in your body's fat cells, are essential because we can't manufacture them in our bodies and so must obtain them from our diet. They provide energy, and help to build cell membranes and other important substances in the body such as hormones.

Our body requires both saturated fats (the type available from butter and coconut oil) and also unsaturated fats (present in olive and other plant oils and fish oil). Omega-6 fatty acids, available in sunflower and soya oil, are plentiful in most Western diets, because they are present in processed foods, but we're now beginning to understand that it's the omega-3 fatty acids that lower inflammation, and that high levels of omega-6 fatty acids can cause oxidative damage to your cell membranes. Nevertheless, the American government still recommends high levels of omega-6 fatty acids. The recommendation of the National Institute of Medicine of the US National Academy of Science of a 10 to 1 ratio of omega-6 to omega-3 fatty acids is weighted too much towards omega-6: other countries, including the UK's Department of Health, suggest a 4:1, 3:1 or even a 1:1 ratio. And fish is given only a minor role on the plate, even though it's a vital contributor of omega-3 fatty acids.

Israel, with one of the highest ratios of omega-6 to omega-3s (20–32:1, compared to the US and UK ratios of 12–20:1), also has the highest incidence of heart disease, type 2 diabetes, cancer and obesity in the world, according to American public health scientists Alice and Fred Ottoboni.[9]

A quick guide to fats

There are two types of fats: saturated fats and unsaturated fats, which differ only in the bond between the atoms, but have vastly different effects on the body.

⇨ **Saturated fats**, made from a bond of a single carbon atom, are mostly from animal foods, but are also found in tropical oils such as palm and coconut oils. The saturated fats in our diets are generally derived from four types: stearic (animal fat and chocolate); lauric (coconut oil); palmitic (palm oil, animal products and dairy); and myristic (coconut oil and dairy).

⇨ **Unsaturated fats** come in two forms: monounsaturated fats (with one double carbon bond between atoms) and polyunsaturated fats (two double bonds). **Monounsaturated** fats are found in olive, rapeseed and canola oils, cashews, peanuts, macadamia nuts, almonds and avocados. **Polyunsaturated** fats include omega-3 and omega-6 fatty acids, described separately below.

⇨ **Omega-3 fatty acids** come from fatty fish such as salmon, mackerel, herring, sardines, and also flaxseeds. They comprise alpha-linolenic acid (ALA), found in flaxseed, and eicosapentaenoic acid (EPA) and docosahexaenoic acid (DHA) (found in plankton and fatty fish).

⇨ **Omega-6 fatty acids** are found in corn, safflower, sunflower, soya bean and sesame oils. They include linoleic acid (LA) and gamma-linolenic acid (GLA), both of which are converted in the body into prostaglandins, which perform many vital bodily functions.

⇨ The evidence now suggests that excess omega-6s bring about chronic inflammation in the body, leading to a plethora of diseases, including heart disease, while omega-3 fatty acids lower inflammation.

⇨ **Trans fats** are formed when an oil goes through a process called hydrogenation, which makes it more solid. This type of fat, known as hydrogenated fat, used for frying or as an ingredient in processed foods, has been shown to damage health (*see page 57 for more information*).

Mistake 4: Both plates include a surprisingly small amount of protein

With the opposition to animal fats and rise of vegetarianism, there's been a relative decline in protein intake as a proportion of all calories consumed – from around 14 per cent of total energy intake in the 1960s to 12 per cent nowadays.

The current recommendations are that protein should account for little more than one-fifth to one-fourth of our total caloric intake. This decision may reflect fat phobia, as many sources of protein (such as red meat) also contain high levels of saturated fat. But while some epidemiological studies (those that study health and disease in particular populations) have implicated excess protein consumption in a raft of degenerative diseases, a similar number of studies have not, making the evidence inconclusive.

In the past, most (73 per cent) hunter-gatherer communities worldwide consumed up to 65 per cent of their energy from animal fat, with a correspondingly small proportion of plant-based carbohydrates (as low as 22 per cent).[10] And while their fat intakes were comparable to or higher than the typical rate of current consumption in Western societies, the type and balance of fats in these subsistence-level peoples were very unlike what we eat in our modern-day diets. In less-developed communities, protein is invariably eaten along with its fat, as the vitamins A and D contained in that fat optimize the uptake and use of the protein.

But today the quality of protein sources is judged only by their total fat content, so that we're asked to make 'lean', 'low-fat' or 'fat-free' choices. The current recommendations don't take adequate account of the essential need for certain fats from these food sources and for vitamin B12, available in only limited amounts in plant foods. Neither animals nor plants can make B12: animals have to get it from what they eat, while for plants to acquire it they must be contaminated by micro-organisms that make the vitamin or have it added to them through, say, fermentation.

Healthy traditional plates

The Weston A. Price Foundation has studied a variety of native cultures with negligible levels of heart disease. All share 10 common characteristics including:

⇨ **Higher animal-protein intake** from meat, fish, eggs and dairy products than recommended in the US and UK governments' plates (up to 35 per cent of daily food)

⇨ **Far greater fish and dairy consumption** than both plates, resulting in four times the calcium and other minerals, and 10 times the intake of vitamins A, D and K2 (although the dairy consumed was whole 'raw' milk, unpasteurized and non-homogenized)

⇨ **Much higher fat intake** (30–80 per cent of total diet) than both plates, but most of it saturated. Just 4 per cent of calories come from polyunsaturated oils naturally occurring in grains, pulses, fish, nuts, animal fats and vegetables

⇨ **Near-equal amounts of omega-6 and omega-3 essential fatty acids (EFAs)**

⇨ **Much higher consumption of raw foods**, including raw meat and fish

⇨ **About half of calories from plants** (fruits, vegetables, nuts and seeds)

⇨ **Some animal bones,** usually from gelatine-rich broth

⇨ **Seeds and nuts, and grains** that are sprouted, soaked, fermented or naturally leavened to neutralize some of the constituent parts, such as phytic acid, that interfere with digestion.[11]

Mistake 5: Carbohydrates (grains, fruits and vegetables) make up 60–80 per cent of a day's intake of calories, with more than a third most likely to be highly processed grain products

Numerous studies show that a high carbohydrate intake – even when less than the proportion suggested in the two plates – is unhealthy.[12]

Mistake 6: All carbohydrates are lumped together

Refined carbs such as sugar and the other 'white stuff' like white flour, white rice and all processed baked goods are considered as 'good' as wholemeal foods and brown rice. The plates' guidelines allow half our grain requirement to be refined. But while the unprocessed carbs consumed in non-industrialized parts of the world contain the nutrients necessary to build lean body tissue, the body has to exhaust its stores of vitamins and minerals like chromium and zinc, which are already deficient in most people, just to metabolize refined carbohydrates.

Refined fructose, which has found its way into an ever-increasing number of manufactured foods in various forms, including high-fructose corn syrup, has proved in studies to be particularly pernicious.[13] A high intake of refined carbohydrates can upset the body's glucose and insulin levels. It's well accepted that refined carbohydrates, which are high on the glycaemic index (see Chapter 9), are rapidly converted into glucose, triggering high levels of insulin that, in turn, cause unused calories to lay down more body fat while raising cholesterol levels.[14] Eating a lot of refined carbs is an established cause of glucose intolerance and diabetes.

Mistake 7: The plates endorse foods damaging to good health

The current UK guidelines allow a full 10 per cent of the day's calories to come from refined sugar, a known and accepted cause of obesity, cancer and diabetes – in fact, of most of the degenerative diseases of modern times.

'Heart-healthy' diets

Over the years, many experts such as California heart specialist Dean Ornish and the late scientist Nathan Pritikin, founder of the Pritikin Longevity Center in Santa Monica, California, have pioneered diets that involve drastically reducing intakes of animal fats and proteins, and sugar (the Ornish diet is a full-on vegetarian diet), plus forbidding oils and foods such as avocados and olives, as well as refined carbs, full-fat dairy and whole eggs. Only 20 per cent of calories on the Pritikin plan, for example, come from fats and proteins; the remaining 80 per cent are derived from complex carbohydrates. And all heart diets recommend avoiding egg yolks: indeed, according to Ornish's spectrum of nutrition, egg yolks are among the least healthful foods you can eat.[15]

But new research shows that, far from being bad for the heart, eggs are among the richest sources of antioxidants, which protect against heart disease. Two raw egg yolks have twice as many antioxidants as an apple and around the same as 25g of cranberries.[16] They can even lower high blood pressure. A review of published studies even suggests that healthy people can eat eggs without raising their heart disease risk,[17] while a study from the Harvard School of Public Health has also contributed to the rescue of eggs from the 'bad food' list by finding that eating one egg a day doesn't increase the risk of stroke or heart disease.[18]

Eggs are only potentially dangerous when they're processed, which means that hundreds of processed foods containing powdered egg yolks can damage arterial walls. Molecules of oxygen and cholesterol combine when heated in spray drying, creating 'oxysterols', a form of cholesterol oxidation that makes it potentially 'cytotoxic [dangerous to cells], mutagenic [capable of causing cell mutations], atherogenic, and possibly carcinogenic'.[19] In fact, scrambling eggs exposes their cholesterol to oxygen with heat, creating an abundance of oxysterols.

Eggs are rich in EFAs (essential fatty acids) and contain all eight essential amino acids (the building blocks of high-quality protein) in the closest thing to perfect ratios. High-quality EFAs, notably the omega-3s found in eggs laid by hens fed on greens and insects, or with seaweed in their diet, are scarce in processed Western diets and even in the official diets recommended by the American Heart Association and British Heart Foundation.[20] In fact, organic eggs provide a wealth of the minerals lacking in even organic vegetables and fruits. The sulphur in eggs and the cysteine it generates are not only excellent for detox, but also good antioxidants.[21] And eggs contain eight times more of the enzyme lecithin-cholesterol acyltransferase (LCAT), which can reduce atherosclerosis and cardiovascular risk in general.[22]

Benecol and cholesterol-lowering 'foods'

Besides avoiding eggs and dairy, heart patients have also been encouraged to consume low-fat spreads and, in 1999, two new margarine-like products claiming to lower cholesterol with daily use became available in the UK and USA. These two spreads, Benecol® and Take Control®, contain plant-based esters, which the manufacturers claim reduce cholesterol by inhibiting the uptake of cholesterol in the GI, or gastrointestinal, tract. In 1999, the Food and Drug Administration (FDA) in the USA said they were satisfied with the manufacturers' claim that these products are safe and had no reported adverse effects, and several studies showed beneficial effects on cholesterol too.[23] The benefits seem impressive at first glance. Benecol claims to reduce total cholesterol by up to 10 per cent and LDL cholesterol by 14 per cent in people who eat three servings per day. Similarly, Take Control can lower total cholesterol by an average of 7–10 per cent when taken daily.

Yet these benefits are no more than what anyone can get from eating organic whole foods and taking regular exercise. What's more, dietary changes and exercise produce long-term effects, while plant esters only last as long as you continue to take them. In one study, two weeks after stopping stanol ester (sistostanol) use, the cholesterol levels of participants returned to pretreatment levels.[24] Clearly these products are yet another fruitless attempt to find a magic bullet for heart disease.

Both spreads have been used in Finland since 1995, but whether there are any long-term adverse effects is still not clear. There is already some concern over the pseudo-hormonal effects of these new substances. Indeed, not long before the FDA's approval of the products, a Swedish review made the disturbing observation that 'further studies are required of [their] phyto-oestrogenic and endocrine effects, and [their] effects on growing children, particularly regarding subsequent fertility in boys'.[25] This has not stopped the makers of Benecol from planning an entire range of pre-packaged foods aimed, according to a company spokesman, at 'cholesterol-concerned' people everywhere.

Although all these official diets and targeted products seek to prevent heart disease by lowering fat, they've missed the elephant in the room. At best, high cholesterol is a crude marker of something gone awry, and that something has to do with what we now consider 'food'.

The role of processed food

A number of doctors have come to the conclusion that one of the chief causes of the epidemic of heart disease in the West is the industrialization of our food supply and the production of processed, packaged foods. In the early part of the last century, there was virtually no coronary artery disease – and yet, within 40 years, it had become the main killer in the West. The rise coincided with a major change in the food supply: the rise of the processed-food industry.

In an insightful editorial in the *Journal of Nutritional Medicine* written in 1991 but still highly applicable, nutritional medicine pioneer Dr Stephen Davies considered whether the late 20th-century Western diet is adequate to meet the current challenges of our environment. His point was that people haven't changed much over 40,000 years of evolution whereas, at least in the West, the diet has.[26] In other words, the business of food may be modern and industrial, but our old-fashioned stomach is still designed for a hunter-gatherer lifestyle. In Palaeolithic times, 21 per cent of our total dietary energy came from fat and 34 per cent from protein. The diet also included 45.7g of fibre and a whopping 591mg of cholesterol compared with today's recommended 300mg or so. Today the average man in the UK takes in 37.6 per cent of energy from fat and 14.1 per cent from protein, plus only 24.9g of fibre and 390mg of cholesterol. According to modern medical concepts, with that level of fat intake our early ancestors should have been dropping like flies. Clearly, fat is not the central culprit in our story.

Numerous studies show that when more primitive populations begin to consume a Western diet, they start dying of heart attacks. When a population of Mexican Indians with virtually no heart problems ate a typical Western diet for two months, they dramatically increased their blood fat levels – by 31 per cent.[27] The main difference between what they ate in their traditional diets and what we eat today isn't a question of meat or fat, but of whole foods.

The real culprit seems to be the large-scale adulteration or 'dismembering' of everything we put in our mouths. Davies argues that one of the results of modern agribusiness, with its domestication of animals, birds and fish, is a substantial reduction in the consumption of essential fatty acids (EFAs), now known to be vital to a healthy immune system. 'Intensive livestock farming of pigs and chickens in particular,' he writes, 'where the animals are kept indoors in overcrowded conditions, is associated with nutrient deficiencies of these animals. Food processing and refining techniques further compromise nutrient content, as do intensive farming techniques which result in soil demineralization. The agrochemical and other environmental pollutants find their way into the food chain, and further disrupt the nutrient value of the foods and stress our detoxification … mechanisms.'[28]

In addition, today's meat business makes liberal use of steroids, antibiotics, tranquillizers and betablockers, while the agrochemical industry currently employs pesticides, herbicides, rodenticides, fungicides and nitrate fertilizers.

Current food processing refines wheat and sugar, thereby reducing trace minerals and vitamins. Similar effects result from current storage methods, food irradiation, and the use of some 3,794 food additives, colourings, sweeteners, texture modifiers and preservatives. The refining of sugar increases blood fats and lowers immunity.

In other words, the culprit isn't cholesterol in our diets, but rather the very means we now use to grow, collect, sell and prepare what we put on the table.

|||||||||||||||||||||||||||||||||||||||||

Chapter 5

THE TRUE CAUSES OF HEART DISEASE

Although medicine has been fingering fats as the culprit in heart disease, it's becoming increasingly clear (and now admitted by the medical community) that the true villain is largely our modern diet – specifically, anything that comes in a box with a long shelf life. Increasingly, the scientific research points to two things that are especially lethal to your heart: trans fats and refined sugar.

As Dr John Mansfield noted in his book, *The Six Secrets of Successful Weight Loss*, until the mid-19th century there was little obesity, diabetes or coronary artery disease (CAD). In fact, the very first recorded case of CAD was in 1912. What has changed since then? Very simply, the introduction in the mid-1950s of refined carbohydrates, including refined sugars, white flour and white rice, followed closely by the introduction of fake fats such as margarine.

As Mansfield tells us, 'In the 60-year period from 1910 to 1970, the proportion of traditional animal fat in the American diet decreased from 83 per cent to 62 per cent. Butter consumption plummeted from 18lb (8kg) per person per year to just 4lb (less than 2kg). Over the same period of time, the percentage of dietary vegetable oil in the form of margarine, shortening and refined oils increased 400 per cent … and the consumption of sugar and processed foods increased by about 60 per cent.'

Insulin regulates glucose (sugar) in blood cells and helps to store it in other cells for use as fuel or for future use. Made by the pancreas, insulin is released into the blood when blood glucose levels rise after eating.

The body becomes insulin-resistant when it's so bombarded with sugar and must produce so much insulin that it turns down insulin-receptor activity in an attempt to protect itself from the toxic effects of high insulin levels. As the body stops recognizing insulin, it produces more and more of it to regulate the amount of glucose in the blood. This situation heralds diabetes, when the pancreas can no longer produce enough insulin to control blood glucose levels. Even more worrying, insulin resistance can also lead to all the major degenerative diseases, including heart disease, high blood pressure, stroke and even cancer.

Researchers at the US Centers for Disease Control and Prevention (CDC) discovered a significant link between sugar consumption and heart risk when they analyzed the diets of more than 30,000 Americans. People who eat too much sugar put on weight and even become obese, which, in turn, increases their risk of cardiovascular disease and death.[1] And drinking just one diet drink every day increases the risk of a heart attack or stroke by a whopping 43 per cent, according to a dietary survey by the University of Miami Miller School of Medicine.[2] It has even been suggested that the artificial sweeteners like aspartame used in such drinks are contributing to an increased risk to heart health.[3]

Other factors can also lead to insulin resistance:

⇨ **A diet rich in high glycaemic index (GI) foods or in processed foods:** Processed foods usually have added sugar or refined carbohydrates, all of which quickly convert to excess glucose in the body, which overwhelms the pancreas, undermining its ability to produce adequate insulin to meet the demand.

⇨ **Stress:** This involves being constantly on fight-or-flight alert, increases insulin production to provide energy for a response and also causes the body to crave high GI foods for instant energy as they are quickly converted into sugar. As Marilyn Glenville wrote in her book *Fat Around the Middle* (Kyle Cathie, London, 2006), fatty or sugary foods eaten during bouts of stress usually end up getting deposited around the waistline 'because the fat is close to the liver, where it can most quickly be converted back into energy if needed'. Over time, too much sugar and excessive fat deposits also lead to the body becoming insensitive to insulin.

⇨ **Too little exercise:** The effect of not taking enough exercise is to minimize the body's efficiency in regulating sugar. Boston-based researchers found that just a single bout of exercise increased the rate of glucose uptake by the working skeletal muscles.[4] In fact, any exercise training can help correct insulin resistance by increasing glucose transport and so prevent type 2 diabetes, the end-result of insulin resistance, when the pancreas can no longer generate the insulin necessary to maintain a normal glucose level in your body.

⇨ **Not enough of the mineral chromium:** After studying thousands of patients over many years, UK nutritional pioneer Dr Stephen Davies discovered that, as patients age, their levels of chromium invariably fall, yet adequate amounts are needed for insulin receptors to work. At least 15 controlled trials have shown that increasing levels of chromium in the diet or as supplements to 10 times what's now the average in the standard diet can reduce insulin resistance and normalize blood sugar levels.[5]

A U-turn on causes

Lately, it's been like watching a school of fish or a flock of birds suddenly change direction: in 2014, medicine declared that fats aren't the cause of heart disease after all. The real culprit is actually sugar. It's been hard to pick up a newspaper of late that hasn't been running regular features and helpful lists for readers about the foods that contain 'hidden' sugars, now described as the 'new nicotine'.

One of the first to break rank was Dr James DiNicolantonio from Ithaca, New York, who says we've been 'led down the wrong dietary road for decades' and is now calling for a public health campaign as pervasive and aggressive as the one enjoyed by the low-fats theoreticians to tell the public that carbohydrates and sugars are the true villains.[6]

Quick on his heels were a team of European researchers from the UK and the Netherlands, who took another look at 76 studies involving nearly 650,000 participants, and concluded that there was no evidence to support the current guidelines for preventing heart disease, which encourage high consumption of polyunsaturated fatty acids and low consumption of saturated fats.[7]

If sugar is the villain, how is it causing heart disease? Some researchers are beginning to abandon the idea that LDL is the so-called 'bad' cholesterol. While it may indeed be clogging up our arteries, it's doing so to repair the damage to the artery wall caused by inflammation, which, in turn, is a response to the physiological stress caused by sugar-laden processed foods.

Another culprit: fake fats

Most processed and low-fat foods are deficient in essential fatty acids (EFAs) and can cause an imbalance by lowering 'good' cholesterol while increasing triglycerides, or stored fat cells in your body.[8] Among the most dangerous of these low-fat foods is margarine, made from hydrogenated oils.

Hydrogenation is a process, dating back to 1912, that enables the food industry to use polyunsaturated fats as a food spread, instead of butter and lard. During hydrogenation, oils are heated to a high temperature and hydrogen is sent through them. In the process, synthetic trans fatty acids (TFAs) are produced, but with a different molecular structure from the essential fatty acids normally found in humans and other mammals. The process also creates 'trans isomers' of fatty acids, which chemically resemble saturated fats.[9]

The amount of TFAs in processed foods can range from 5 to 75 per cent of the total fat content. Neither US nor British law requires manufacturers to state the amount of hydrogenated fat in a product, only whether or not it's present. TFAs can have a 'disastrous' effect on the body's ability to use EFAs, says nutrition expert Dr Leo Galland, author of *Superimmunity for Kids* (E.P. Dutton, New York, 1998).

They are even more detrimental when heated, turning into something akin to polymers in plastic. Hydrogenated fats are found in fast food like chips (or fries) and doughnuts, and in the vegetable oils used in shortening and cookies/biscuits. They account for up to 10 per cent of the content of some margarines, although some manufacturers, such as Van den Bergh Foods, which makes Flora, have now stopped hydrogenation entirely.

George V. Mann, a doctor in Nashville, Tennessee, who has researched and written extensively on the subject, argues that lipoprotein receptors in cells are damaged by TFAs. As this impairment prevents the body from processing LDL cholesterol, the body's cells crank up their rate of cholesterol synthesis, eventually leading to high levels of cholesterol in the blood. Indeed, numerous studies show that blood cholesterol is quickly raised in people who consume TFAs.[10]

An eight-year study of 85,000 women by Harvard Medical School found that those eating margarine had an increased risk of coronary heart disease. Hydrogenated vegetable oils have not only failed to provide the expected benefits as a substitute for highly saturated fats, but they've actually 'contributed to the occurrence of coronary heart disease'.[11] The more TFAs you eat (and have stored as body fat), the greater your risk; in fact, one Welsh study showed a strong link between TFAs in body fat and heart-disease fatalities.[12]

When the late Dr Mary Enig, formerly of the chemistry and biochemistry department at the University of Maryland, analyzed the TFA content of some 600 foods, she reckoned that Americans eat between 11 and 28g/day of TFAs – accounting for one-fifth of their total intake of fat.[13] To give you an idea of how this happens, one large portion of chips fried in partially hydrogenated oil contains 8g of TFAs, as does 60g (2.2oz) of processed cheese.

The Harvard study reckoned that TFAs could account for 6 per cent of all deaths from heart disease, or 30,000 deaths a year in the USA alone. And, of course, heart disease rates are high in northern European countries, where consumption of TFAs is high, but low in the Mediterranean countries, where TFA intake is low because the main dietary fat is olive oil.

Our epidemic of heart disease can be directly linked to the introduction of hydrogenated fats in food, with the first major outbreak recorded in 1920. Before the First World War, when cheese and butter were dietary staples, death from coronary thrombosis was rare. At least three studies have shown that the incidence of heart disease fell during times when countries stopped consuming margarine and returned to butter (such as during the Second World War).

Yet many researchers stubbornly continue to link heart disease to animal fats such as butter. The 2002 final report of the US National Cholesterol Education Program (NCEP) recommended soft and TFA-free margarines over butter,[14] and the influential EURAMIC study, which covered eight European countries and Israel, claims it was also unable to find any definitive link between margarine and heart problems, although the authors did admit to a potential connection in populations consuming large quantities of margarine.[15]

Processed meats

New evidence has been pointing to preservatives in processed food as another cause of high blood pressure and hardening of the arteries. Phosphates in processed foods such as processed cheeses and in cola drinks can stimulate the production of fibroblast growth factor 23 (FGF23), a bone-derived hormone that controls sodium and calcium levels in the body. If levels of FGF23 are high, the kidneys have to absorb more calcium, and this leads to hardening or calcification of the arteries. High levels of the hormone also mean high levels of sodium, say researchers at the University of Veterinary Medicine Vienna in Austria.[16] People with kidney disease have raised levels of FGF23 and sodium, a situation that leads to cardiovascular problems.

Processed meats have also been linked to heart failure, particularly in men. For every 50g (1¾oz) of processed meat (the equivalent of, for example, one slice of ham) eaten every day, the risk of death from heart failure rises by 38 per cent. Heavy eaters of processed meat are twice as likely to die of heart failure as men who eat small amounts of such meats infrequently.[17]

The role of stress

Besides dietary issues, a major international investigation, the Interheart study, discovered that 'persistent severe stress' increases the risk of heart attack by two and a half times.[18]

While all of us suffer stress from time to time (such as when we're rushing to catch a train or to meet a work deadline), the type that leads to heart disease is the chronic variety, when we feel powerless and socially isolated, with no end in sight to the problem.

Dr Malcolm Kendrick, author of *The Great Cholesterol Con: The Truth About What Really Causes Heart Disease and How to Avoid It* (John Blake Publishing, London, 2008), has listed the types of stress he thinks cause heart disease, and the main ones, in his view, include:

⇨ Bullying bosses

⇨ Racism

⇨ Long-term money worries

⇨ Poor social network and feeling 'dislocated' from others

⇨ Unloving or abusive partner.

Other markers of heart disease

While medicine focuses on total, LDL and HDL cholesterol as the primary markers of heart disease, other factors may be just as important, especially now that cardiovascular disease is better understood as an inflammatory process.

Even conservative groups like the American Heart Association (AHA) are recognizing the role of inflammation in heart disease, and several studies have confirmed the association. Inflammation is the body's immune response to stress and infection. In medicine, the concept of stress refers to any 'insult' to the body, such as a poor diet of 'fast' and processed foods or exposure to environmental pollutants, as well as tension and depression, or feeling alone, isolated and helpless.

One study found that the root of the problem was not cholesterol so much as the blood-clotting factor fibrinogen, a protein marker of increased inflammation. Those who had high levels of both fibrinogen and LDL cholesterol were six times more likely to have cardiovascular disease. Conversely, people with low fibrinogen levels rarely go on to develop heart disease, even when their LDL levels are high.[19] Men with fibrinogen levels in the top third were more than twice as likely to suffer from heart disease as those in the bottom third. And smokers seem to have high levels of fibrinogen, which confirms the long-held concerns about a link between smoking and heart attacks.

C-reactive protein

If heart disease truly is a disease of fat accumulation, as the cholesterol hypothesis suggests, then levels of liver-synthesized C-reactive protein (CRP) shouldn't be able to accurately predict future heart problems – and yet they do, according to some reports. A marker of increased inflammation, CRP levels are also highly accurate predictors of stroke, diabetes, heart attack and cardiovascular death even years before the event.[20] Statin drugs appear to have the unintended benefit of lowering CRP levels, and patients with lower levels recover better from heart disease – even in cases where the drug fails to reduce LDL cholesterol.[21] This again points to the importance of inflammation. In a study comparing 506 men who had suffered a heart attack with 1,025 healthy controls, inflammation was a significant indicator of heart disease. Men with the highest levels of CRP in their blood were more than twice as likely to suffer from the condition.[22]

Homocysteine

New research indicates that cardiovascular risk may be increased by homocysteine, an amino acid found in higher levels in patients who have suffered strokes or other heart conditions. Its pathological involvement was first identified back in 1969, when extraordinarily high levels of homocysteine were found *post mortem* in patients suffering from arteriosclerosis.[23] Yet the link with arterial lesions was dismissed and put down to rare metabolic effects among these particular subjects.

Later, however, a review of 27 studies of homocysteine and vascular disease by the University of Washington confirmed that homocysteine was a strong predictor of heart attack risk and carotid artery obstruction. The authors concluded that a 5μmol/L (micromoles per litre) increase in homocysteine raised the risk of coronary artery disease as much as a 1.1mmol/L (millimoles per litre) or 19.8mg/dL (milligrams per decilitre) increase in cholesterol.[24] In fact, the biggest ever heart health investigation, the US Framingham Heart Study, revealed that the higher the level of blood homocysteine, the greater the likelihood of carotid artery narrowing (stenosis).[25]

The influential Harvard-based Physicians' Health Study of nearly 15,000 male doctors similarly found that the men with the highest homocysteine levels were three times more likely to have a heart attack than those with the lowest levels,[26] while a study from Bergen in Norway found a graded relationship between homocysteine blood levels and overall death rates. Coronary artery disease patients with levels above 20μmol/L were nearly five times more likely to die than those with levels below 9μmol/L.[27]

This amino acid is the by-product of the normal breakdown of proteins in the body. The European Concerted Action Project on homocysteine and vascular disease, involving 750 cases and 800 controls from 22 collaborators across Europe, but based in London, concluded that homocysteine interacts with lipid factors like cholesterol and triglycerides, and substantially increases the risk of heart disease even when cholesterol is normal or low.[28]

Gum disease: the missing link

Gum disease, or 'periodontal disease', apart from being unattractive and uncomfortable, can also raise the risk of heart disease and stroke.

Researchers at Seoul National University College of Dentistry in South Korea discovered that people with an advanced form of gum disease – or 'periodontitis' – have a higher risk of ischaemic stroke (the type caused by a blood clot) than people with diabetes, and around the same risk as people with high blood pressure. Both high blood pressure and diabetes are well-recognized risk factors of ischaemic stroke. Research involving 265 hospitalized, non-fatal, ischaemic stroke cases and 214 non-stroke controls found that those with periodontitis – characterized by inflammation and infection affecting not just the gums, but also the ligaments and bones that support the teeth – were four times more likely to have suffered a stroke, which was double the risk posed by diabetes.[29]

As Dr Nigel Carter, Chief Executive of the British Dental Health Foundation, pointed out, 'This research is significant because it helps to quantify the importance of oral health compared to other risk factors. The findings are startling. The fact that high blood pressure carries a similar risk to gum disease is in itself a significant finding. The other finding, which shows that gum disease nearly doubles the risk of non-fatal strokes compared to diabetes, is totally unexpected.'[30]

But this wasn't the first study to find a significant connection between gum disease and stroke. In 2004, German researchers at the University of Heidelberg studied 771 men and women, 303 of whom had recently had an ischaemic stroke. They found that, among men and younger (under 60) participants, severe periodontitis increased the risk of stroke more than fourfold. Gingivitis (gum inflammation), a milder form of gum disease, also raised the risk of ischaemic stroke, while tooth cavities didn't.[31] An earlier study, by Harvard School of Dental Medicine researchers, followed over 41,000 men for 12 years and showed that those with gum disease and fewer teeth (tooth loss is a common consequence of untreated gum disease) were significantly more likely to suffer a stroke.[32] A handful of other studies have reported similar findings.

In addition, periodontal disease has been linked to artherosclerosis – the hardening and narrowing of the arteries. In one small Italian study, people with carotid artery plaques (fatty deposits) had significantly poorer gum health than those without plaques – even after taking into consideration other established cardiovascular risk factors.[33] What's more, a review of 31 published reports found an association between gum disease and atherosclerosis, heart attack and cardiovascular disease.[34] Clearly, there's a connection between the health of our gums and the health of our heart.

The perio-cardio link

Although some may argue that the state of our gums is merely a reflection of our overall health, there are several plausible theories as to how gum disease might cause heart disease and stroke. One suggests that oral bacteria could affect the heart by entering the bloodstream and attaching to fatty plaques in the coronary arteries, so contributing to the formation of blood clots.[35] Clots can obstruct normal blood flow, restricting the delivery of nutrients and oxygen that the heart needs to function properly.

Another hypothesis has to do, again, with inflammation – the body's inbuilt reaction to infection. Researchers suspect that gum disease may not just cause inflammation in the mouth but may, over time, also contribute to systemic inflammation, now known to play a crucial role in a wide range of diseases not usually considered inflammatory, such as cardiovascular disease. Indeed, the inflammation theory may explain why periodontal disease has also been linked to other systemic disorders such as diabetes,[36] rheumatoid arthritis,[37] Alzheimer's disease[38] and chronic kidney disease.[39]

In further support of this hypothesis, an Italian study has discovered that treating gum disease can have beneficial effects for the rest of the body. When the researchers examined the carotid arteries of 35 people who had mild to moderate gum disease but were otherwise healthy, they found high levels of inflammatory markers before treatment. A year after treatment, they found significantly lower levels of oral bacteria and thickening of blood vessel walls associated with atherosclerosis.[40]

Nutritional factors

Another possibility is that gum disease and heart disease are both consequences of a poor diet and nutrient deficiencies. This would explain the link between gum disease and other systemic disorders. Coenzyme Q10 (CoQ10), for example, is a vitamin-like enzyme found in practically every cell of the body – and not having enough has been linked to both periodontitis and heart disease. CoQ10 participates in cell energy production, and makes cell membranes more resistant to oxygen damage. It's abundant in the heart mostly because of the huge energy requirements of cardiac cells.

Studies suggest that up to 96 per cent of people with gum disease may have below-normal levels of CoQ10.[41] There's also evidence that supplementing with CoQ10 has beneficial effects on oral health. In one study, presented at the 63rd Meeting of the Vitamin Society of Japan in Hiroshima in 2011, 45 patients with mild to moderate gum disease were given either ubiquinol (150mg/day; an active form of CoQ10) or a placebo for two months. At the end of the study, the ubiquinol group showed statistically significant improvement in dental plaque adhesion and bleeding gums.

In another double-blind trial, 18 patients with periodontal disease took either 50mg/day of CoQ10 or a placebo for three weeks. All eight of those taking CoQ10 saw an improvement, compared with only three of the 10 taking the placebo.[42]

Vitamin C deficiency has also been linked to both gum disease and heart disease. One study of Finnish and Russian men found that those with periodontitis were more likely to have low blood levels of vitamin C. The researchers pointed out that 'vitamin C deficiency is also an independent risk factor for myocardial infarction', and noted the need for more studies to explore the relationships between vitamin C deficiency, gum disease and cardiovascular disease.[43]

Other research suggests that vitamin C might be a useful treatment for gum disease. When people with periodontitis who normally consumed only 20–35mg/day of vitamin C were given an additional 70mg/day, their gum health improved in just six weeks.[44]

Omega-3 fatty acids may also play a role in the health of our gums. A recent study from Harvard discovered that higher dietary intakes of docosahexaenoic acid (DHA) and, to a lesser degree, eicosapentaenoic acid (EPA), were associated with a lower prevalence of periodontitis in more than 9,000 adults across the USA.[45] Omega-3 fats are well known for their anti-inflammatory properties and beneficial role in heart health. It could well be that a deficiency of omega-3 fatty acids in the diet contributes to the link between gum and heart health.

Possible causes of high blood pressure

Many cases of high blood pressure seem to be caused by one or more of three major culprits:

⇨ **Inflammation:** Researchers from Harvard Medical School have found high levels of C-reactive protein (CRP), an indicator of inflammation, in the blood samples of 5,365 women with hypertension.[46]

⇨ **Prescription drugs:** Many prescription drugs can cause hypertension, including NSAID (non-steroidal anti-inflammatory drug) painkillers, which can double the risk of high blood pressure in people 65 or older.[47] Ironically, antihypertensive drugs themselves can increase blood pressure. In 945 hypertensive patients, 16 per cent saw their blood pressure levels rise even higher while taking one of the four major blood pressure-lowering therapies – namely, diuretics, calcium-channel blockers, beta blockers and ACE inhibitors.[48]

⇨ **Stress:** The stress of modern life can raise blood pressure, as can arguments and loud noises. Even the constant sounds of traffic can do it, as found by researchers in Stockholm, Sweden. Around half the city's residents with hypertension live within 100 metres (109 yards) of a busy road. On comparing their medical conditions with people living in quieter neighbourhoods, the researchers reckoned that traffic noise can increase high blood pressure risk.

this was never commercially available because it caused tumours, muscle deterioration and death in laboratory dogs (reactions still seen in people taking mevastatin's modern equivalents), it nevertheless caught the attention of America's drug giant Merck (MSD outside the USA). By 1978, Merck scientists had isolated lovastatin from a different fungus (*Aspergillus terreus*).

Merck now had a solution, but no problem – since what did cholesterol have to do with heart disease anyway? Although a few scientists had mooted the possibility of an association, most heart physicians weren't buying it.

So Merck put its PR machine into overdrive and decided to bypass doctors and go directly to the public. It began a heart health campaign, explaining that we have two types of cholesterol: 'good' HDL (high-density lipoprotein); and 'bad' LDL (low-density lipoprotein), which builds up in arterial walls and eventually leads to heart attack. The good sort could keep the bad in check, they reasoned, and in addition to a good diet and plenty of exercise, statin drugs were a great way to help achieve a healthy cholesterol balance.

The facts, though, weren't supportive of the PR drive. At around the time Merck's spin doctors – and soon those of other drug companies too – were telling the public about their bad cholesterol, the Framingham Heart Study was reporting that people over the age of 50 were more likely to die of cardiovascular disease if their cholesterol levels were decreasing.[3]

This surprising association was repeated years later when researchers looked at elderly Japanese American men (71–93 years of age) participating in the Honolulu Heart Program in Hawaii.

Those who had consistently low cholesterol levels at examinations 20 years apart were 1.6 times more likely to die than those with higher levels. 'Long-term persistence of low cholesterol concentration actually increases the risk of death,' they concluded.[4]

No proof of benefit

As other researchers have also discovered, cholesterol is vital for healthy bodily functioning. It influences energy, immunity, fat metabolism, thyroid activity, liver synthesis, stress tolerance, adrenal function and – increasingly as we age – brain function. High cholesterol levels may even protect against heart-related deaths in people over the age of 50.[5]

And if cholesterol is important for overall health, then it's perhaps not surprising to find that statins – which lower cholesterol levels – don't in fact help us to live longer.

Irish researchers in their trawl of the published literature could find no studies to prove conclusively that statins add years to our lives. What they did find was that men aged 69 and older didn't live longer and didn't have fewer heart attacks.

Some studies even suggested that statins could hasten death. The drugs triple the risk of coronary artery calcification, when calcium settles in arterial walls – a problem usually associated with high cholesterol (which the statins supposedly lower). But medicine's best-kept secret was the Illuminate trial, which was stopped early after statins were found to actually increase the risk of both cardiovascular and non-cardiovascular adverse events (such as infections and cancer).[6]

The Galway researchers also found evidence that statins increased the risk of diabetes, cataract formation and muscle weakness (myopathy) that could last for 12 months, as well as acute kidney failure, liver dysfunction, erectile dysfunction and immunosuppression.

A heart-healthy enzyme

As we've seen in Chapter 1 and intermittently throughout this book, cholesterol is important for overall health. However, so too is coenzyme Q10 (CoQ10), which supplies energy to cells (*see page 158*). It's also important for maintaining muscle strength, especially those of the heart. CoQ10 and cholesterol share the same pathways, so when you interfere with cholesterol production in the liver, you also affect CoQ10.

If low levels of CoQ10 cause heart failure, and statins block the production of this enzyme, this may explain why statins are associated with heart disease. The link has been known for years and, at one stage, Merck applied for a patent to add CoQ10 to its statins, although this was never acted upon.

Statins aren't entirely without merit. Middle-aged men with pre-existing heart conditions – specifically, coronary artery disease – seem to be better off taking the drugs, but that's about it. For the rest of us, they don't protect against heart disease, but might even bring it on, along with a range of other side-effects.

Quite a testament for the bestselling drugs of all time.

Tick-box meds

In many cases, drugs aren't needed for any specific complaint but are prescribed simply because the patient is elderly – a phenomenon that's been described as 'tick-box medicine'. One example is bringing down levels of blood cholesterol, especially in the elderly. Yet this is clearly a failure to understand the changing metabolism in older patients, who appear to need higher levels of cholesterol for their general wellbeing and, especially, mental sharpness.

As mentioned above, men in the Honolulu Heart Program aged 71 to 93 showed that those with the lowest cholesterol levels – 2.09–4.32mmol/L (37.62–77.76mg/dL) – were up to 40 per cent more likely to die than those with higher cholesterol levels. The study, which measured cholesterol changes over 20 years, questioned whether there was any 'scientific justification for attempts to lower cholesterol to concentrations below 4.65mmol/L [83.7mg/dL] in elderly people'.[7]

Not only can higher cholesterol levels be beneficial in the elderly, but the cholesterol-lowering drugs themselves may be doing more harm than good, according to a study by Yale University. While these drugs provided a marginal benefit for reducing heart-related death, patients over 70 died of other causes as a result of taking them.[8]

In the early 1990s, a number of large-scale studies revealed that patients on low-cholesterol diets or drugs were more likely to die violent deaths, including accidents and suicide, than those eating a regular diet.[9] This bizarre connection was dismissed as a quirk until it was confirmed by a number of subsequent international studies. Research from Italy confirmed that low cholesterol levels do indeed seem to make people suicidal. When the blood cholesterol levels of 300 people who'd attempted suicide were compared with those of a matching group of people who'd never tried to harm themselves, in virtually all cases the suicidal group had lower levels of cholesterol at around the time of their attempts.[10]

Link to low serotonin

In 1992, Dr Hyman Engelberg, at the Department of Medicine at Cedars-Sinai Medical Center in Los Angeles, proposed that the increase in violent deaths seen with lower levels of cholesterol might actually be due to low serotonin.[11] One of the functions of this brain hormone is to suppress harmful behavioural impulses like aggression. As Engelberg concluded, 'A lowered serum cholesterol concentration may contribute to a decrease in brain serotonin, with poor suppression of aggressive behaviour.'

This idea is supported by several clinical trials showing a connection between low cholesterol and depression, especially in men over age 70. In a study from the University of California at San Diego (UCSD), the authors concluded that the findings were 'compatible with observations that very low total cholesterol may be related to suicide and violent death'.[12]

Interestingly, one effect of a newer class of antidepressant drugs – the selective serotonin reuptake inhibitors (SSRIs), including fluoxetine (Prozac) – is to block serotonin from reaching certain cells in the nervous system. Numerous instances of violent and suicidal tendencies among patients taking these drugs have been reported. The UCSD team found that depression was three times more common in patients aged over 70 with low blood cholesterol than in those with higher levels. They also found that the extent of depression correlated with cholesterol: the lower the cholesterol, the more depressed the patient.

Serotonin and tryptophan

The problem described above may affect only older age groups, as there's never been any evidence of a link between violence and cholesterol-lowering drugs in younger people. However, there's evidence that people on weight-loss programmes have significantly lower blood levels of tryptophan – the essential amino acid from which serotonin is derived – as well as significant changes in serotonin levels.[13] We get tryptophan from specific foods, mainly proteins, as well as dietary supplements. Comparisons of the dietary habits of populations in different countries reveal that people with low tryptophan intakes do indeed have higher rates of suicide. Also, patients who are severely depressed have low tryptophan levels and feel even worse when on low-tryptophan diets; but as their depression improves, so do their levels of tryptophan.[14]

'They almost ruined my life'

But these days the statin net has spread even further: virtually every healthy man aged 60 and every woman over 65 is now eligible to start taking these cholesterol-lowering drugs under the new UK 'best practice' guidelines. Previously, only those with high cholesterol counts – and so, according to the theory, at greater risk of heart disease – were in line to take these popular drugs.

Underlying this radical change of policy by the UK National Institute for Health and Care Excellence (NICE) is the belief that statins don't have any serious side-effects. Conveniently, just before the NICE announcement was made, researchers from Imperial College London claimed just this after reanalyzing 14 trials involving 46,262 patients.[15]

In one UK national newspaper, the study inspired the headline, 'Statins have no side-effects,' suggesting that anyone who complained of one must be hysterical, attention-seeking or just plain wrong.

Try saying that to Mary Stamp, 67, who suffered badly from the drug's two most common side-effects: muscle weakness and cognitive decline. It all started around 2007 when she went with her friends for a blood test while in Cyprus, where she has her second home.

The test revealed high cholesterol levels, and the Cypriot doctor put her on atorvastatin (Lipitor). On her return to the UK, her usual doctor was happy to continue the prescription, but she began to notice feeling a little weak. 'I just thought I had caught flu,' Mary recalled, 'but I also thought it must be because I was starting to get old.'

This went on for several years until she was unable to get out of bed. This couldn't just be old age, she thought: after all, she was a keen walker and swimmer, and she ate a healthy vegetarian diet. She started to research her symptoms and thought that perhaps the statin had something to do with it. So she stopped taking the drug and her symptoms disappeared.

Even then, she wasn't entirely sure if the statin was to blame, so when a year later her doctor prescribed simvastatin, she started taking that instead. Again, she started to suffer twinges and pains, but the serious side-effects began only after 18 months, when one day her body completely seized up, which she said was 'terrifying'. If the drug was doing this to her muscles, what was it doing to her heart?

The drug was also interfering with her brain and cognitive abilities. As a retired holistic sports therapist, Mary had always prided herself on her mental acuity and general intelligence, but suddenly she was losing it, and in worrying ways.

One day she looked at a measuring jug and couldn't understand what the measuring lines signified; another day she had to call out a mechanic because she couldn't make her car go, only to be told that the automatic gear was still in 'park'. On another occasion she booked the same flight to Cyprus twice. Sometimes she just couldn't remember words, and she also wasn't able to sleep. 'I really thought this was dementia,' she said, 'and that I was losing my mind.'

As she has private medical insurance, Mary insisted on having a full neurological examination. And again suspecting the drug, she stopped the simvastatin, so that, by the time she took the battery of tests, the neurologist could find nothing wrong with her. She'd passed all the tests with flying colours and was her old self again.

Today, she's an anti-statin ambassador and tells her story to everyone she can. Her husband is her latest convert, and in 2015 he refused to start statin therapy.

She admits there are plenty of people who have been on statins for years and never suffered any ill effects. But then there are the others who, like herself, thought they were suffering from dementia and blamed it on their advancing years.

So don't tell Mary there are no side-effects with statins. To control her high cholesterol levels – a problem she believes she inherited – she eats healthily and well, and avoids all junk food and processed sugars.

The bottom line with statins

Cholesterol-lowering statins are one of the great 'lifestyle drugs' of our times. Zocor (simvastatin) can be bought at your local pharmacy in the UK without a prescription, and so good are they for all of us that they could even be added to the public water supply, says Dr John Reckless, chairman of Heart UK.

Such exuberance, and prolific prescribing by doctors, have made statins the world's most profitable drug family, with annual sales of around $26 billion (£17 billion). Most doctors see statins as the perfect drug, a life-saver with virtually no side-effects. Unfortunately, the data support neither of these claims.

Just one group of people appear to benefit from statins: men who've had a previous heart attack. Healthy men and women will not see their life expectancy improved whatsoever, even if they've taken a statin every day for five *years*. Although early Scandinavian Simvastatin Survival Study (4S) initially found that statins can achieve between a 66 per cent reduction in overall mortality per year,[16] and a 22 per cent reduction in overall mortality,[17] eventually it was discovered that the manufacturer of the statin Zetia (ezetimibe) withheld data until it was pressed to reveal its findings by the US Congress. This concealed evidence showed that the drug was ineffective.[18]

Common problems encountered when taking these drugs include muscle tenderness and weakness, or myopathy. One statin, cerivastatin (Baycol), was taken off the market because it was found to cause this debilitating muscle condition – with the result that 31 people even died while taking it.

These drugs can also cause Parkinson's, a disease of the central nervous system. In one study, statin users who developed Parkinson's had levels of LDL cholesterol three times lower than average, suggesting that very low levels of cholesterol may play a role in the development of the disease.[19]

If you think you need a statin ...

If you must take a statin drug, and you are part of that small population of men who could benefit from it, consider taking the smallest dose possible. New evidence shows that even the recommended daily dose of 40mg/day causes muscle pain and potentially fatal muscle weakness, leading to a complete breakdown of muscle tissue.[20] Higher doses, or taking the drug with other drugs, has a magnifying effect, causing a far higher incidence of myopathy than claimed by the official figures.

Statins can also lead to memory loss, depression, confusion, irritability and dizziness, and major birth defects of a scale not seen since the thalidomide scandal. There's also growing concern that they can cause cancer and heart failure too.[21]

||||||||||||||||||||||||||||||||||||||||||||||

Chapter 7

OTHER HEART DRUGS

Heart attack, or myocardial infarction, is defined as the 'death' of heart muscle tissue caused by an inadequate blood supply. It can be brought about in one of two ways. Usually it's caused by obstruction of a coronary artery because of atherosclerosis (fatty plaques), or it may happen suddenly or after a history of angina pectoris (heart-related chest pain caused by lack of oxygen to the heart). For those people who show little evidence of blockages, as many do, it's assumed that a spasm of the coronary artery may be responsible. To treat these two possible causes, patients are offered a range of drugs to unclog and/or dilate the arteries by thinning the blood or boosting the strength of the heart in pumping blood.

Ironically, the symptoms of angina may not always lead to heart disease. Instead, believe it or not, they can lead to an increased resistance to heart attack.[1]

Two amazing adaptive changes generally occur within the heart muscle after a brief attack when there's insufficient oxygen for the heart to function.[2] One is the development of alternative blood vessels through which enough blood flow can be maintained,[3] while the other is a more general protective and strengthening effect on the heart.[4] Observations of these adaptations are well established, although not well understood, and many complex theories have been proposed to explain them.[5]

This doesn't mean we should stop treating angina, since even with treatment this natural protective adaptation takes place. And it also doesn't mean we should stop worrying about heart disease because, in half of cases, your first heart attack is your last. The real question is how best to treat these conditions, as the conventional approach is rather hit or miss.

Beta blockers

Beta blockers, which are supposed to lower blood pressure and stabilize the heart's rhythmic action, only reduce the possibility of a further heart attack by a very small margin, while causing other undesirable side-effects such as dizziness, impotence, nausea, cold extremities, nightmares and insomnia. And the latest evidence from the New York University School of Medicine, which tracked 44,708 heart disease patients for more than three years, discovered that the drugs don't protect heart patients. Those taking the drugs are just as likely as those not taking the drugs to have a second heart attack or stroke. In fact, in those with heart-disease risk factors, there were more cardiovascular disease-related deaths among people taking beta blockers.[6]

Beta blockers can also bring about sudden irregular or abnormal heartbeats (arrhythmias) that can be fatal, while also being asymptomatic. In fact, not having symptoms of arrhythmia is much more commonly seen than symptomatic cases – in a ratio of 12 to one.[7] A 2000 editorial in the *Journal of the American*

College of Cardiology accompanying the report of this halted trial concluded that all antiarrhythmic drugs may be considered potentially lethal.

Calcium-channel blockers

This family of antihypertensive drugs, including verapamil, diltiazem and nifedipine, can also stop blood from coagulating (clotting). Unfortunately, what's good for the heart isn't necessarily good for the stomach. This class of drugs can cause severe stomach bleeding in the elderly.[8] The US Food and Drug Administration (FDA) has also cautioned against using nifedipine, as this agent has been shown to create first a sharp drop, followed five hours later by a sharp rise, in blood pressure, thus increasing the risk of heart attack.[9]

Antiarrhythmics

These drugs can cause the very problem they're trying to treat: a heart with irregular beats. In one large trial, there were significant numbers of deaths associated with encainide and flecainide. Almost 6 per cent of patients died of arrhythmias while taking these drugs compared with 2 per cent taking a placebo. Similarly, around 2 per cent died of a heart attack or heart failure compared with 0.7 per cent of the placebo group.[10] Once again, those not taking the prescribed drugs had better survival rates after heart-related incidents.

Another trial of an antiarrhythmic agent was stopped early because the death rate due to arrhythmias was unacceptably high.[11]

Nitroglycerin

This agent, the main ingredient in dynamite, has been routinely given as an emergency spray or pill to hospital patients with chest pain (angina pectoris) since 1867, but has never been tested for safety. When researchers at Stanford University School of Medicine finally did so in a rat model, they found that the drug increased the risk of heart attack, especially when given continuously by intravenous drip. It damages heart tissue and suppresses aldehyde dehydrogenase 2 (ALDH2), an enzyme that mops up free radicals and protects the heart against injury when blood flow is restricted – such as during a heart attack. In general, the drug doubled the size of the heart attack after being given continuously for 16 hours.[12]

Failed foxglove

One of the most commonly prescribed drugs for heart failure is digitalis (digoxin), derived from the foxglove plant, even though its long-term benefits and safety have never been proven.

The latest evidence suggested it may protect against death in those who are already at high risk because of chronic heart failure. Nevertheless, after 200 years of usage, the Digitalis Investigation Group thought it was about time to do a proper study of the agent. They gave 3,397 heart patients 0.25mg/day of digoxin and 3,403 patients a placebo; all participants were also given diuretics and ACE inhibitors. After an average of 37 months, there were 1,016 heart-related deaths with digoxin and 1,004 with the placebo. The only crumb of comfort was that those taking the drug had 3 per cent fewer hospitalizations.[13]

Another study, carried out by Kaiser Permanente Northern California, found higher death rates in both men and women whose systolic heart failure – where the left ventricle becomes enlarged, thin-walled and floppy, and so unable to pump blood properly – had been treated with digoxin for two and a half years.[14]

Antithrombotics

Another popular method in medicine is thrombolytic therapy, also known as 'fibrinolytic therapy', which uses clot-busting drugs to clear blood vessels. In an investigation of 1,050 patients given angioplasty, a procedure that involves inflating blocked arteries (as described in Chapter 8), compared with those treated with thrombolysis in a group admitted to hospitals in Seattle, Washington, the risk of death was 5.6 per cent with thrombolysis and 5.5 per cent with angioplasty.[15] For the same result, the use of drugs was less traumatic and less expensive too.

The greatest risks occur in the 24 hours after treatment. A review of nine studies found deaths were more likely to occur during the day of or day following treatment, especially among the elderly or those patients waiting at least 12 hours after experiencing symptoms before they started to seek treatment.[16]

Antibiotics

These agents are sometimes used on the basis of the theory that the respiratory virus *Chlamydia pneumoniae* plays a part in furring up the arteries: the antibiotic kills the virus, so stopping the furring.

In fact, antibiotic treatment does nothing to stop atherosclerosis, as two major studies have discovered. The first involved over 4,000 patients with coronary artery disease given either the antibiotic azithromycin or a placebo; the second recruited a similar number of patients with acute coronary syndrome who were given either the antibiotic gatifloxacin or a placebo. In neither trial did the antibiotic group fare any better than the placebo group – and neither antibiotic reduced the occurrence of cardiovascular events despite long-term treatment.[17]

Although the virus has been detected in around 40 per cent of atherosclerotic plaques, and mice and rabbits inoculated with the virus have developed inflammatory lesions in arteries, the bottom line is that the majority of heart patients don't have the virus, and animal trials are not always an indication of similar activity in humans (not to mention being sometimes needlessly cruel and pointless). And, in any case, the fact that the virus is present in some plaques doesn't mean there's a causal link between the two.

Could a heart attack be good for you?

Some doctors in Germany and Britain say that, contrary to expectation, a heart attack may in certain circumstances be beneficial. To prove it, they deliberately induced heart attacks in patients with heart blockages, or 'hypertrophic obstructive cardiomyopathy'. Of the 18 patients on whom they've tried this technique, 16 showed major improvement in their symptoms afterwards. The blockages were cleared by the attack, leading to better blood flow in the left ventricular outflow tract and a slight increase in exercise capacity.[18]

Combination heart drugs

Most doctors think that if one drug does some good, two will do twice as much good. The beta blocker/calcium-channel blocker combination has been very popular for patients with heart disease. The thinking behind it is that a low dose of both drugs will decrease the number and severity of angina attacks more effectively than a high dose of either drug alone, and with fewer side-effects. As many factors like age or state of overall health influence the balance between the supply of oxygen to the heart and its demand for oxygen, and a single drug can address only some of these factors, doctors have assumed that a second heart drug with different actions might work in a complementary fashion. Because drugs for angina often have rebound circulatory effects (the same symptoms return after stopping the drug), another assumption has been that these unwanted effects may be counteracted by a second drug.

But these two assumptions have never stood up to scientific scrutiny. According to one review of controlled clinical trials, combining a calcium-channel blocker with a low-dose beta blocker has rarely had any additional benefits for angina patients, and may even increase adverse reactions by up to 60 per cent.[19]

The other problem is that most doctors don't really understand how each drug relieves angina on its own. Beta blockers work by blocking the heart's chemical stress receptors, so inhibiting the rise in heart rate and blood pressure during exertion (stress), leading to the assumption that these drugs relieve angina and other symptoms of coronary artery disease by decreasing the heart's oxygen demands.

In contrast, since electrical impulses from the heart (which control its contraction and relaxation with every heartbeat) involve calcium ion signalling, calcium-channel blockers – which slow these signals down – can theoretically also slow the heart rate. They also relax arteries, thereby increasing blood flow and supposedly easing how hard the heart has to work to pump blood throughout the body. Consequently, many doctors have assumed that these drugs relieve blocked blood vessels by increasing the oxygen supply to the heart through the extra blood reaching that organ.

So the notion that calcium-channel blockers and beta blockers work in tandem to increase heart oxygen supply and lower oxygen demand is the rationale offered by the medical community for their combined use.

In fact, both drugs alleviate angina through strikingly similar mechanisms – reducing heart oxygen use, limiting heart rate increases and relaxing blood vessels. And recent observations show that the two drugs don't necessarily interact well together. Although calcium-channel blockers can stop arterial constriction in the heart, which is caused by beta blockers, this may only happen where blood flow is normal. Likewise, while beta blockers may prevent the rapid heart rate induced by calcium-channel blockers, this may not prevent the decrease in blood pressure frequently caused by those drugs and may even worsen angina if blood pressure falls markedly. Beta blockers can boost the blood pressure-lowering effect of calcium-channel blockers and so increase the risk of a diminished blood supply to the heart. In many other ways, the two drugs work antagonistically.

The combination can also make angina worse if the two drugs combine to cause rapid heartbeats. Beta blockers can also cancel out the ability of calcium-channel blockers to relax the blood vessels. Abnormally low blood pressure causing dizziness and sudden falls, worsened heart failure with abnormally slow heart rates and conduction defects (that is, problems in getting electrical instructions from the brain) may occur more often with the combination of the two drugs than with single-drug therapy. The drugs in combination also hamper the ability of the heart to pump.

The author of a report on these problems, Dr Milton Packer of the Division of Cardiology at Mount Sinai School of Medicine in New York, also warns that, of all the calcium-channel blockers drugs, verapamil (sold as Cordilox, Securon SR, Verelan, Covera-HS, Isoptin) is the most likely to interact unfavourably with beta blockers. Besides inhibiting heart contraction, the combination could dangerously impair the sympathetic nervous system's control of your blood supply and also enhance the effect of beta blockers in less than desirable ways. The combination may also slow the elimination of the drugs from the body, so making any adverse effects even worse.

Drugs for hypertension

Any 'abnormal' blood pressure reading – and especially any level above 140/90mmHg – will almost inevitably trigger a prescription for an antihypertensive drug.

As with heart attack and angina, the medical treatment of hypertension involves a vast litany of drugs that rarely help a condition that can often be resolved by judicious diet and exercise. Some drugs, meant to cure hypertension, can actually exacerbate the condition, while others can kill you. Beta blockers, diuretics, reserpine, methyldopa and clonidine are usually prescribed for hypertension, yet all have been implicated in various other disorders, such as depression, impotence and sexual dysfunction, loss of appetite, nausea and tiredness. One particularly worrisome effect is postural hypotension – a sudden drop in blood pressure on standing – which can then cause dizziness and falls. Given this risk factor, it's not surprising that hypertensive drugs are a major cause of hip fractures among senior citizens.[20]

A study of 2,000 patients with high blood pressure from 13 general practices across England revealed that only just over half of those taking antihypertensive drugs had achieved moderately healthy blood pressure levels.[21] Even the modest goal set by the US Third National Health and Nutrition Examination Survey (NHANES III) of less than 140/90mmHg was reached by only 27 per cent patients, despite the drugs.[22] Excluding the USA, a survey of more than 18,000 patients in 26 countries worldwide found that only a third of patients managed to achieve the blood pressure targets set by their doctors.[23]

Traditionally, a diuretic (water pill) has been the doctor's first line of defence against hypertension. But this supposedly 'safe' drug has been shown to cause a 32 per cent greater risk of diabetes compared with a placebo or a beta blocker.[24]

European 'best practice' guidelines recommend that 'more than one drug is needed' particularly for patients with blood pressure at the high end of normal and a history of cerebrovascular, cardiovascular or peripheral artery disease.[25] The four most common two-drug therapies combine a diuretic with a calcium-channel blocker, a beta blocker, an ACE inhibitor or an angiotensin-receptor blocker.

But the combination of a diuretic and calcium-channel blocker can dramatically increase the risk of a heart attack. In a study of 335 hypertensive patients, taking a calcium-channel blocker with or without a diuretic increased their risk of heart attack by 60 per cent. A similar figure was seen in a group of 384 patients taking a calcium-channel blocker with a beta blocker.[26] But in yet another study, researchers from the University of Washington in Seattle estimated that the risk was even higher: taking a calcium-channel blocker with a diuretic nearly doubles the likelihood of having a heart attack.[27]

Beta blockers are hardly any better. They increase the risk of stroke – but not heart attack – and don't lower blood pressure, according to a major review of studies involving more than 100,000 patients.[28] In the UK, the British Hypertension Society was so concerned by these findings that it changed its 'best practice' guidelines in 2006, removing beta blockers as a first-line treatment for hypertension, even though these drugs are still regularly used as such elsewhere in the world.

ACE inhibitors are generally not well tolerated and cause a range of side-effects – from hypotension (too low blood pressure), heart attack, hepatitis and jaundice to mental confusion, acute kidney failure and impotence.

And while angiotensin-receptor blockers were designed as safer alternatives, studies suggest they're every bit as dangerous as ACE inhibitors. Valsartan can increase the risk of heart attack by 19 per cent, while candesartan, another angiotensin-receptor blocker, causes a 36 per cent increase in heart attacks.[29] And despite spending $26 billion (£17 billion) a year globally on drugs with a dubious safety record – and which may not even work very well – doctors could instead prescribe the old-fashioned diuretics and get the same results, but without the even greater risks posed by these newer drugs. When 42 studies involving nearly 200,000 patients with high blood pressure were analyzed, low-dose diuretics worked just as well as any of the newer agents (beta blockers, calcium-channel blockers, ACE inhibitors and angiotensin-receptor blockers).[30]

Most drugs are not only vastly overused, but largely unnecessary for most mild cases of raised blood pressure. One study found that almost half the patients over 50 had normal blood pressure levels a year after stopping their drugs. According to Professor Peter Sever, an expert on high blood pressure at Imperial College London, GPs delude themselves into thinking they are treating blood pressure effectively. 'Their big decision is taken,' he points out, 'when they decide whether or not to start therapy, but once they've started their patients on a drug, they appear very reluctant to change.'

While there isn't much evidence that antihypertensive drugs do a lot of good, there's plenty to show they do great harm.

Beta killers

Not only is there only moderate evidence for antihypertensives actually working, but other evidence for beta blockers suggests they can be a killer. Their potential for harm came to light only after they were being given regularly to all patients undergoing surgery – including non-heart surgery – to reduce stress on the heart.

The practice, adopted across Europe in 2009, was based on fabricated data and research. The falsifications, perpetrated by

Don Poldermans, formerly professor of cardiology at the Erasmus Medical Centre in Rotterdam and former chairman of the European Society of Cardiology (ESC) guidelines committee, were uncovered in 2011.

In the two intervening years, hospital surgical patients given beta blockers were 27 per cent more likely to die from any cause within 30 days, while the risk of stroke or hypotension was increased, according to researchers from Imperial College London.[31] Two of this study's authors, cardiology professor Darrel Francis and research fellow in cardiology Graham Cole, estimated that the practice has killed 800,000 people across Europe, including 10,000 Britons, according to an article in *The Sunday Times* (26 January 2014). This piece also appeared on the *European Heart Journal* website, but was removed within hours. Defending the action, the journal's editor Thomas Lüscher said that publishing Francis and Cole's estimates had been a mistake: 'This issue is complex and should not be handled like that,' he stated. 'Such statements are not scientifically valid and create panic among patients and physicians, and in this form are not only completely inappropriate but ethically questionable.'[32]

Drugs that cause hypertension

A large number of drugs for treating completely different conditions can actually cause hypertension:

⇨ **Cyclosporine**, a powerful immunosuppressant, which can raise systolic blood pressure[33] and lead to arterial hypertension in heart and kidney transplant patients[34] in as little as a few weeks[35]

⇨ **Oral contraceptives**[36]

⇨ **Hydrocortisone**, at least in men aged 22–34 years[37]

⇨ **Non-steroidal anti-inflammatory drugs (NSAIDs)**, especially in the elderly[38]

⇨ **Tricyclic antidepressants**, taken for panic disorders[39]

⇨ **Nasal decongestants and cough syrup**, if taken in large enough doses.[40]

Drugs for stroke

Much of the research on drugs for stroke is focused on finding the single most effective preventative for strokes, the most popular options being anticoagulants, antiplatelets, antihypertensives, diuretics and surgery. Typically, treatment ends up being a combination of any or all of these. It's also important to note that the term 'effective' in stroke research generally means 'cost-effective', as prevention is usually aimed at reducing the number of patients requiring hospitalization and treatment for stroke, rather than improving their quality of life.[41]

Women in particular are at risk of stroke from an increased number of medical causes. For example, it's long been known that the Pill increases the likelihood of stroke, with even low doses of oestrogen (less than 50mcg) raising the risk of blood clots by as much as four times.[42] Hormone replacement therapy can also be risky. Although the reports are mixed, it's clear that women, especially those with cardiovascular disease, run a greater risk of developing rare but lethal torsades de pointes (ventricular tachychardia), an abnormal heart rhythm; the culprit seems to be female sex hormones, particularly oestrogen.[43] There also seems a gender bias towards men in the early diagnosis and treatment of heart disease, as they have always been (wrongly) considered at higher risk. Although there are some differences in the ways that cardiovascular disease manifests in women, when they receive care it's often inappropriately the same as is offered to men.[44]

Drugs that can cause strokes

Various types of categories of drugs and substances can cause cerebral haemorrhages, leading to stroke. If you're at risk of this condition, you could do well to avoid the following:

⇨ **Sumatripan**, the migraine drug[45]

⇨ **Beta blockers**[46]

⇨ **Nifedipine**, a calcium-channel blocker[47]

⇨ **Chemotherapy**, or the hormones given during chemotherapy[48]

⇨ **Hormone treatments** like HRT and the Pill[49]

⇨ **Oral anticoagulant therapy**[50]

⇨ **Nasal decongestants**, used to excess[51]

⇨ **Blood pressure-lowering drugs**[52]

⇨ **Phenylpropanolamine**, present in many over-the-counter weight loss drugs, nasal decongestants and cold preparations[53]

⇨ **Recreational drugs** like ecstasy, cocaine and methamphetamines[54]

⇨ **Anabolic steroids**[55]

Clot-thinning medications for stroke and thrombosis can also lead to strokes. These include:

⇨ **Streptokinase/subcutaneous heparin therapy**, combination therapy[56] and recombinant tissue-type plasminogen activators (rt-PAs)[57]

⇨ **Anticoagulant medication**[58]

Stroke can also be brought on by:

⇨ **Ingesting hydrogen peroxide**[59]

⇨ **Lumbar myelography**, a radiographic examination of the spine usually using a contrast dye[60]

⇨ **Heavy alcohol consumption** in men.[61]

Blood-thinning that leads to stroke

When thrombolysis, the use of drugs to dissolve blood clots, is performed after cerebral infarction, the likely result is another stroke – this time caused by cerebral haemorrhage. Warfarin, one of the standard blood-thinning drugs, doubles the risk of stroke within the first seven days. People with irregular heartbeats (arrhythmias) are at special risk, with a 2.3 times greater chance of stroke by usually the third day after starting the drug.

The risk continues over the first month, but is lower after the first week, say researchers at McGill University in Montreal, who made the discovery after looking at more than 70,000 people taking the anticoagulant. Of these, 5,519 people, or 2 per cent, suffered a stroke after starting treatment.

Although the drug stops blood from clotting by suppressing the body's production of vitamin K, the researchers believe it may have a contrary effect in the first few days by actually making the blood 'stickier'.

In people with arrhythmias, the heart doesn't pump efficiently, making the blood more likely to clot in any case, and warfarin only seems to make this worse: clots that break away and travel to the brain can cause stroke.[62] Other evidence suggests warfarin could be causing excessive bleeding in patients with atrial fibrillation (irregular or fast heartbeat), the other class of patients prescribed this drug.[63]

Heparin and warfarin are both indicated for cerebral haemorrhage, but there's an ongoing debate over the use of agents such as streptokinase (SK) and rt-PA. Three large SK trials were terminated early because of high death rates due to intracerebral haemorrhage.[64]

Thrombolysis is a high-risk strategy for stroke, especially if administered 'late' (three to six hours after the event). The National Institutes of Neurological Disorders and Stroke (NINDS) trial showed an even smaller 'therapeutic window' (less than three hours) for the administration of rt-PA.[65] The Multicentre Acute Stroke Trial–Italy (MAST–I) was one of those abandoned due to high death rates. Risk of mortality significantly increased more than threefold in those taking SK plus aspirin.[66]

The MAST–I results were clearly not unique, and the effects of different thrombolytic drugs may vary depending on the drug and how it's given.[67] As always, it's the elderly – the majority of stroke patients – who are more likely to experience cerebral haemorrhage and die as a result.[68]

Aspirin to treat strokes

The 'magic bullet' philosophy underlying modern medicine does nothing to help stroke patients. Perhaps the best example of this is the wholesale administration of aspirin as a treatment and preventative for stroke. Aspirin not only thins the blood, but also lowers blood pressure. This means it's recommended not only as prevention but also as treatment, for patients with constricted blood vessels and those who've suffered heart attacks or transient ischaemic attacks (TIAs) – minor strokes of short duration. The fact that aspirin is cheap, readily available and familiar to patients is also in its favour.

Evidence to support aspirin for strokes has been accumulating for years. But the supposedly definitive thumbs-up came from the Antiplatelet Trialists' Collaboration (ATC) in a series of articles published in 1994.[69] The conclusions echoed many of the ATC's earlier findings.[70] Even though these findings were, on closer inspection, more circumspect than acknowledged at the time, aspirin was quickly hailed as the conquering hero of stroke treatment and it's since been prescribed widely (almost recklessly) throughout the world.

But the side-effects of high-dose aspirin as prescribed for stroke treatment are debilitating and sometimes fatal. Aspirin is usually prescribed in doses of 75–325mg/day. Although lower than the mega-doses of 1–4g/day seen 15 years ago, this is still not without risk. Dyspepsia (stomach upset, nausea and vomiting) is seen in 10 to 20 per cent of cases.[71] More seriously, using data from the 1990 Nurses' Health Study, there is a 43 per cent risk of gastrointestinal bleeding with regular aspirin use (more than two 325mg tablets a week), rising to 77 per cent with six to 14 tablets a week. The risk was strongly related to how much you were taking, not how long you'd taken it.[72]

There's continuing debate over the optimal time frame for aspirin therapy.[73] Certainly, long-term use can cause serious side-effects. Aspirin may slow blood-clotting, but it can also deplete the body of certain essential vitamins and minerals, especially iron. Not surprisingly, one of the effects of long-term aspirin therapy is anaemia, which can complicate haemorrhagic disorders. Other adverse effects include ulcers (particularly in the elderly), liver damage and allergic reactions such as hives, wheezing, tinnitus, chronic catarrh, headache, confusion and, more rarely, abnormally low blood pressure followed by collapse. Asthmatics can die from severe attacks brought on by an aspirin.

A new, and more dangerous, drug

Designed to prevent stroke in patients with atrial fibrillation, the anticoagulant Pradaxa (dabigatran) quickly became a blockbuster, generating more than $1 billion (£658 million) in annual sales after being approved by America's drugs regulator, the Food and Drug Administration (FDA), in 2010, and by the European Medicines Agency a year later. Unlike warfarin, the anticoagulant of choice for more than 60 years, dabigatran required no monitoring of patients. Excited by the drug's potential for massive cost savings, the FDA gave its approval after just one major study, when usually it requires two. But in 2011, just a year after its approval in the USA, dabigatran was already being cited as the most dangerous prescription drug available, having received 179,855 reports of 'serious, disabling, and fatal adverse drug events,' up 9.4 per cent from 2010. Warfarin, its main competitor, accounted for 72 deaths at the time.[74]

In 2012, the UK's National Institute for Health and Care Excellence (NICE) and similar groups in the USA, Canada and throughout Europe responsible for setting healthcare standards endorsed the drug for routine heart care. But within a few weeks of this acceptance, it all started to unravel. In May 2014, Boehringer Ingelheim (BI), dabigatran's manufacturer, had to pay out $650 million (£428 million) in lawsuits to settle 4,000 cases of harm or death associated with the drug. Yet, at the time of writing, doctors are still prescribing dabigatran. Neither the regulators nor the manufacturer have decided to take it off the market, despite the number of deaths and serious injury it's caused. The circle has been broken yet again.

Drugs that can cause heart disease

Heart patients are often advised to take NSAIDs (non-steroid anti-inflammatory drugs) to help ward off another attack … but this advice isn't just wrong, it may actually be lethal.[75]

If you're taking the UK's most popular painkillers, you could be increasing your risk of a fatal heart attack – especially if you already have a heart condition or diabetes. Prescription and over-the-counter (OTC) painkillers containing diclofenac can boost your chances of a heart attack by 40 per cent, a risk only slightly below that associated with the painkiller Vioxx (rofecoxib); (*see page 110*). Although the risk is greater for prescription diclofenac, the OTC version can still increase your chances of a fatal heart attack – and the risk increases with the dose.

Diclofenac is an NSAID, a category that includes some of the most common drugs around, including aspirin and ibuprofen. Used in prescription and OTC painkillers such as Diclofex, Diclomax, Dyloject, Flamrase, Motifene, Rhumalgan and Voltaren, it's usually taken to ease the pain of arthritis, toothache, back sprains and migraine. It also reduces fevers, and is often taken for flu symptoms and premenstrual pain.

Not surprisingly, it's the UK's most commonly prescribed painkiller, with more than six million prescriptions written for it every year.

More heart problems

Until 10 years ago, doctors believed that the only major problem with NSAIDs was the risk of gastrointestinal problems such as stomach bleeding, but this all started to change when studies began to suggest that NSAIDs in general – and Vioxx in particular – caused heart problems.

By 2004, the evidence was overwhelming, and Merck, the manufacturer of Vioxx, was finally forced to take it off the market. Although the true figures may never be known, it's been estimated that around 60,000 died from a heart attack and 140,000 suffered serious heart problems while taking the drug.

The following year, Pfizer took its own painkiller Bextra (valdecoxib) off the market because of similar concerns. Like Vioxx, Bextra increased the risk of heart attack and stroke, and also caused a skin rash that was fatal in some cases. Also, people who'd undergone heart surgery were more than twice as likely to suffer a stroke or heart attack if taking Bextra.

Vioxx was a special type of NSAID, a COX-2 inhibitor, designed to relieve pain, but without the stomach problems associated with aspirin and the other usual NSAIDs.

So, were the heart risks only prompted by the COX-2 inhibitors? Researchers decided to find out by assessing the risks of the entire NSAID family. Patricia McGettigan, at Hull York Medical School, and David Henry, at the Institute for Clinical Evaluative Sciences in Toronto, Canada, took another look at major studies of NSAIDs, involving a whopping more than 2.7 million people, with an eye on potential heart risks.

Not surprisingly, Vioxx came out on top as the one most likely to cause heart problems, with an increased overall risk of 45 per cent. But what did surprise the researchers was that diclofenac ran a close second, with a 40 per cent higher risk. Even low doses of diclofenac – such as typically found in OTC products – increased the heart attack risk by at least 22 per cent.

Ibuprofen, another OTC painkiller, increased risk by 18 per cent, but only if you took more than 1,200mg/day – which is easily achieved if you take just three high-dose 400mg tablets. Overdosing with amounts greater than 1,200mg makes ibuprofen one of the most lethal NSAIDs and raises heart-attack risk by 78 per cent. In contrast, naproxen has a 9 per cent risk that remains constant no matter how much you overdose.[76]

Patients most at risk

What are the implications of these results for your health? According to McGettigan, while young healthy people who take these drugs don't have much to worry about, those with an already increased risk of heart problems do: 'A patient with previous heart problems, high blood pressure and diabetes,' she explained, 'has an annual background risk of heart attack of over 5 per cent. Use of diclofenac will increase that by 40 per cent, giving an annual risk of over 7 per cent. In other words, one in 50 such patients might suffer an avoidable heart attack.

'In contrast, a healthy young woman has an annual risk of heart attack of less than 0.1 per cent – she will experience a negligible increase in cardiovascular risk with any of the commonly used NSAIDs.'

The risk with some NSAIDs for people with heart problems was highlighted in a study published in *Circulation*, the official journal of the American Heart Association. The study analyzed data from nearly 84,000 heart attack survivors, 42 per cent of whom were taking a prescription NSAID. The researchers, from Copenhagen University Hospital in Gentofte, found that even short-term treatment with most NSAIDs was associated with an increased risk of death and repeat heart attacks.

Diclofenac was associated with the highest risk. Those taking the drug were more than three times more likely to suffer another heart attack within a week of the first. As the researchers concluded, 'Neither short- nor long-term treatment with NSAIDs is advised in this population, and any NSAID use should be limited from a cardiovascular safety point of view.'[77]

Yet another study, this time of patients with coronary heart disease and high blood pressure in the USA, found that NSAIDs dramatically increased the risk of death, heart attack and stroke.[78]

Efficacy *vs* safety

The evidence linking the commonly used NSAIDs with heart risks is now undeniable, the risks posed by diclofenac and Arcoxia (etoricoxib) being particularly worrying. Ultimately, the research so far highlights the serious failure of the drugs 'watchdogs' to protect public health while underscoring the importance of adequately assessing drug safety by carrying out proper clinical trials.

To avoid yet another Vioxx disaster, establishing the safety as well as the effectiveness of all NSAIDs should be a top priority.

Another Vioxx?

Drugs giant Merck (MSD outside of the USA) was finally forced to pull its bestseller painkilling COX-2 inhibitor drug Vioxx after the evidence that it was causing fatal attacks became overwhelming. This made a big dent in the company's revenues: in 2003, the year before the drug was withdrawn, Vioxx was achieving sales of $2.5 billion (£1.6 billion) a year.

Merck was quick to respond. It started to push another NSAID painkiller, Arcoxia (etoricoxib), which was soon approved in more than 70 countries, including the UK. But one country refused to allow it onto the market: the USA.

The US Food and Drug Administration (FDA) asked Merck for more safety information because it feared the drug would have risks similar to those of Vioxx. And the FDA was right to be concerned: Arcoxia has exactly the same risk profile as Vioxx.

In other words, it too increases the risk of fatal heart attack by 45 per cent.

Antacids

NSAIDs are not the only OTC remedies to pose risks to your heart. Antacids, those mild OTC remedies for indigestion, increase your risk of pneumonia by up to three times and, as one study has shown, pneumonia can increase the risk of heart attack and stroke fivefold.[79] The study found an association between respiratory infections, like bronchitis and pneumonia, and heart attack and stroke. The risk was five times greater within the first three days of getting the infection, and then subsided over the following weeks.

As stated by one of the lead study researchers, Professor Patrick Vallance, at the London School of Hygiene and Tropical Medicine: 'After the age of 50, we all have some degree of furring up in the arteries, but most of the time it sits there fairly harmlessly. However, during infection, stable deposits become unstable and may break off, causing blockages that may lead to a heart attack or stroke.'

Antacid compounds reduce gastric acid secretion, so allowing bacteria and viruses to make their way into the respiratory tract. These, in turn, can cause pneumonia, which leads to inflammation that destabilizes fat deposits around the arteries, sometimes causing a heart attack or stroke. Yet who would connect this with the antacid they'd taken several weeks before?

Antidepressants

There's another class of drug to avoid if you have heart disease. They increase the chances of heart attack and stroke by speeding up the ageing process of arteries, making them thicker and more rigid.

All members of the antidepressant drug family, including SSRIs (selective serotonin reuptake inhibitors), cause thickening of the arteries, say researchers from Emory University's Rollins School of Public Health. In a study of 513 middle-aged male twins, the researchers found that those taking an antidepressant had arteries markedly thicker than those not taking the drug. Overall, the added thickness was equivalent to what's usually seen in someone four years older. In the 59 twin pairs followed for 13 years, the carotid artery in the twin taking SSRIs like fluoxetine (Prozac) was thicker by a factor of four compared with the twin not taking the drug.[80]

Antibiotics

Clarithromycin, an antibiotic taken by millions of people every year to treat bacterial infections, can increase the risk of fatal heart attack. It affects the heart's electrical activity, and it's this mechanism that's thought to increase the risk of fatal heart rhythms. Researchers estimate that the drug increases such a risk by 76 per cent compared with penicillin V, an antibiotic with no known heart effects. In absolute terms, clarithromycin could cause 37 cardiac deaths per one million courses of treatment, say Danish researchers.[81]

Azithromycin – another antibiotic marketed as Zithromax, or Z-Pak – is at its most lethal in the first five days of starting treatment when, compared with amoxicillin, the risk of death linked to cardiovascular disease has been shown to be increased by 2.5 times. The risk was highest for those who already had heart disease, with 245 additional heart deaths per one million courses.[82]

Heart-risky NSAIDs

All of the following drugs can cause or aggravate heart problems and might be best avoided:

⇨ diclofenac (Voltaren, Anuva, Diclon, Clofast)

⇨ etodolac (Lodine, Etopan)

⇨ etoricoxib (Arcoxia)

⇨ ibuprofen (Advil, Nurofen)

⇨ indomethacin (Indocin, Indocid)

⇨ meloxicam (Movalis, Melox)

Heart drugs: dangers at a glance

The following drugs commonly prescribed for heart problems can cause a range of major side-effects:

⇨ **Vasodilators** (nitrates, calcium-channel blockers): Can cause headaches, dizziness, hypotension (abnormally low blood pressure) and potentially fatal altered heartbeats (either too fast or too slow); calcium-channel blockers can also cause constipation, vomiting, oedema, sudden rapid heartbeat, liver disorders, rashes, depression and gastrointestinal disorders.

⇨ **Antihypertensives** (ACE inhibitors, diuretics, potassium-channel blockers): ACE inhibitors can cause sudden drops in blood pressure, dangerous rises in potassium, fluid in the lungs (when used with some diuretics), kidney dysfunction, muscle cramps, diarrhoea, nausea, fatigue, rashes, abdominal pain, heart palpitations, jaundice, sleep disturbances, mood swings and impotence. Diuretics can cause gastrointestinal disturbances, dry mouth, skin rashes, photosensitivity, kidney damage and pancreatitis. Potassium-channel blockers may adversely affect your thyroid, alter the electrical rhythms of the heart, lead to visual problems or liver damage, sensitize the skin to light and damage the lungs.

⇨ **Beta blockers:** May cause potentially fatal slowing of the heartbeat, asthma, fatigue, cold hands and feet, sleep disturbances, nightmares, stomach upsets and rashes.

⇨ **Antiarrhythmics:** Run the risk of heart failure, chest pain, choking sensations, light-headedness, impaired vision, skin discoloration, phototoxicity, diarrhoea, fever, lupus-like symptoms, psychosis and liver damage.

⇨ **Antiplatelets (aspirin, anticoagulants):** Can lead to gastrointestinal problems, respiratory disorders, stroke, diarrhoea, vomiting, throbbing headaches and hypotension.

⇨ **Cholesterol-lowering drugs:** May cause severe depression, suicidal and/or violent tendencies, constipation, vitamin K deficiency, impotence, and there's an established link too with cancer of the lung, thyroid, testis and lymph nodes.

Chapter 8

OPERATIONS FOR HEART DISEASE

The operation was successful, but the patient died. That's how bypass surgery began in 1962, when renowned American cardiac surgeon David Sabiston, chairman of the department of surgery at Duke University School of Medicine, in North Carolina, grafted a vein, taken from the patient's leg, and attached it to the ascending aorta to bypass a blocked right coronary artery during open-heart surgery.

Sabiston was gratified when the graft took – indeed, more gratified than his patient, who died just three days later due to 'unrelated complications'.

Despite such inauspicious beginnings, some 50 years later heart bypass surgery – or a coronary artery bypass graft (CABG), as doctors call it – is among the most frequently performed surgical operations, with some 500,000 carried out in the USA every year and around 20,000 (first-time) operations in England and Wales. Around 10 per cent of all heart patients will eventually undergo a coronary bypass, especially if they have one or more coronary arteries that are either blocked or severely narrowed.

There's no doubt that it's miracle surgery for some, but besides being a common reason for patients to go under the knife, the coronary bypass is also one of the most unnecessary of operations. Heart surgeons have suspected this since the 1970s, when several major studies revealed that bypass surgery did not improve survival except among patients with severe coronary artery disease, especially of the left ventricle.

Even though it's an appropriate treatment for a small minority of coronary artery disease sufferers, the bypass seems to be surviving better than its patients. Perhaps this is not surprising when you consider that, in the USA, it's one of the most lucrative of all surgical procedures, with surgeons earning about $100,000 (£66,000) an operation. This means the treatment is costing Americans an average of $500 billion (£329 billion) a year to treat just 500,000 people.

How a bypass works

During the operation, the surgeon removes veins from the patient's leg, forearm or chest, and grafts these onto a healthy portion of one of the main coronary arteries to get around the portion that's blocked. The traditional, or 'on-pump', method is carried out while the heart is stopped, and the patient and his blood supply are attached to a pump, which oxygenates the blood and pumps it back into the patient.

However, because of the large potential for things to go wrong with this method, surgeons are increasingly opting for the 'off-pump' technique, also known as 'beating-heart bypass surgery', where the heart is kept going and stabilized by special equipment – a procedure that surgeons maintain is far safer.

Balloon angioplasty

Since 1978, balloon angioplasty has superseded bypass surgery as the less invasive way to prevent a heart attack in patients with clogged coronary arteries. The procedure involves threading a tiny balloon catheter into the blocked or stenosed (narrowed) artery and inflating it. This will clear the vessel, usually by smashing the fatty plaques against the arterial wall. After this is done and the balloon catheter removed, a tiny piece of metal scaffolding called a 'stent' is usually inserted to hold the artery open. Simply put, the entire process is a bit like clearing a blocked drain.

What doctors tell you about bypass and angioplasty

Doctors tend to advise bypass rather than angioplasty if you're in any of the following situations:

⇨ All three arteries of the heart are blocked or narrowed (or two arteries if you have diabetes, which affects circulation)

⇨ Your left main coronary artery is very narrow

⇨ You need to repair or replace a heart valve anyway

⇨ Your heart is no longer pumping efficiently.

The received wisdom has been that angioplasty is the safer option – that is, until a recent US National Institutes of Health (NIH) study analyzed the records of around 189,000 patients and found that, after four years, the CABG group (or 'cabbages', as many doctors privately refer to them) had a mortality rate of 16 per cent compared with 21 per cent with angioplasty.[1]

What doctors *don't* tell you about bypass and angioplasty

Doctors will insist that bypass and angioplasty are indispensable treatments, but they often don't tell you the downsides:

⇨ **You could be recommended for unnecessary surgery based on a faulty test** Computed tomography (CT) angiography, which is fast replacing the standard stress test in doctors' surgeries, uses intravenous dyes and CT scanning technology to provide an 'inside view' of the coronary arteries. The older stress test uses a gym bike or running machine, followed by a simple check of heart function.

The problem is that the new CT-angio test is doubling the rate of invasive cardiac procedures, including surgery, researchers at Stanford University School of Medicine have discovered. Lead researcher Mark Hlatky wonders just how many of these invasive procedures are necessary. 'If you pull a 75-year-old off the street and give him this test,' he said, 'it's unlikely the coronary arteries will be completely normal.'[2]

⇨ **There's no big advantage in having angioplasty** In terms of results, the differences between the two operations are small (see the NIH study cited above). When all major studies comparing the two ops are combined, there's no significant difference between the two when it comes to deaths and adverse effects.[3]

In fact, one in 10 heart patients will return to hospital for emergency treatment following angioplasty or a stent procedure. They are also far more likely to die of heart problems in the next 12 months than someone who was treated but didn't need hospital aftercare.

In a survey of 15,498 patients needing hospital care following an intervention, such as angioplasty, nearly 10 per cent had undergone the procedure within the previous 30 days and, of these, 106 (0.68 per cent) died while in hospital.[4]

⇨ **The 'low mortality' of the bypass isn't all that low** According to a review of all major published studies, three out of every 100 people who have the bypass will die, and up to one in four will suffer complications.[5]

What else doctors don't tell you about the bypass

The benefits of bypass surgery are unpredictable and it can even bring on the very problems it was supposed to prevent.

⇨ **It may not make your heart work better:** A review of 37 studies concluded that the patient's heart function improved in only about a third to just under a half of all cases.[6] The rest had basically the same heart function they had before the operation.

⇨ **Your heart may develop abnormal heart rhythms:** More than a quarter of all patients will suffer atrial fibrillation (irregular heart rhythms) after their bypass surgery, despite intravenous magnesium, which is supposed to help prevent it.[7]

⇨ **You could suffer angina:** Although bypass surgery is supposed to eradicate angina, which is usually caused by arterial obstruction, around one in five bypass patients will still suffer heart pain after the surgery.[8]

⇨ **You could have a stroke:** One in six CABG patients has a stroke or some other adverse brain effect, including brain death.[9]

⇨ **You could experience mental decline:** In other words, you could have 'post-perfusion syndrome' as it's officially known, or 'pumphead', as doctors refer to it among themselves. After a year, roughly a third of all CABG patients will suffer some deterioration of their mental faculties,[10] mostly because of the high risk that, as a result of the surgery, thousands of dislodged microscopic blood clots find their way to the brain.[11]

⇨ **You could develop gut problems:** This is the experience of one in every 20 bypass patients.[12]

⇨ **There's a high risk of future breathing difficulties:** More than half of all CABG patients complain of chest pain and breathing difficulties after five years, increasing to nearly 75 per cent of patients after 15 years.[13]

⇨ **The off-pump procedure could cause permanent brain damage:** The procedure carries more than five times the risk compared with on-pump of grafts not taking.[14]

⇨ **You could die within a year:** More than 6 per cent of patients, or one in every 17, die.[15]

⇨ **You're likely to need a repeat op to bypass the original bypass:** Your chances of needing a second surgery increase by around 5 per cent every year.[16]

The bottom line is that most bypass patients will need further surgery within a decade to repair work that was previously done or for first-time work on other vessels.

Dollars and stents

Since 1986, when a cardiac surgeon inserted the first stent into the first 'guinea-pig' heart patient, doctors believed they'd finally cracked the problem of atherosclerosis with the best of modern high-tech medicine.

Balloon angioplasty had been shown to be a blunt instrument, often causing damage to the arterial wall, as well as blood clots. Stents were created ostensibly to solve its limitations after doctors noticed that 'restenosis', or re-narrowing of the artery, occurred within six months in as many as three-quarters of all patients. In many instances, the diameter of the blood vessels treated was only 16 per cent larger than before treatment.

In other words, to solve the problems caused by the high-tech solution, another high-tech solution was born: the stent, a device inserted as a flat-packed piece of mesh tubing and then expanded, ostensibly to keep the 'drain' open and unblocked, and usually helped along by a cocktail of antiplatelet drugs to prevent blood clots.

Although the drug/stent combination appeared to solve the blood-clot problem, it did nothing to prevent arteries furring up: within six months, some 40 per cent of stents were blocked again, requiring a repeat operation.[17]

So the medical device companies came up with yet another solution: coating stents with a thick polymer containing sirolimus, a powerful immunosuppressant agent derived from a *Streptomyces* bacteria species. This agent drip-feeds into the system in low doses – a process called 'elution'– to stop the body's natural attempts to close the artery.

These so-called 'drug-eluting stents' (DES) have their own set of problems. A Swedish study of around 20,000 patients found that deaths and heart attack rates were 30 per cent higher for up to three years among DES patients compared with patients who'd received the old-style 'bare-metal' stents.[18]

A survey of hospitals across the USA also showed that, in nearly a third of cases, stents that were inserted under non-emergency conditions to keep blocked arteries clear are not only unnecessary, but potentially fatal: some of the latest versions of stents are poorly designed and may easily become deformed within the blood vessel.[19]

The case of the shrinking stent

Like an echo of the recent breast cancer implant scandal, some of the latest DES stents suffer from a basic design flaw, causing them to concertina (the stent support rings 'nest' into each other after being inserted). Although first noted by Colm Hanratty and Simon Walsh of the Belfast Health and Social Care Trust, Northern Ireland, in the Promus Element device (made by Boston Scientific), they've since found such deformations in all DES devices.[20]

The Irish researchers detected a higher rate of 'longitudinal stent deformation' (LSD) with the everolimus-eluting Promus Element stent compared with other stents.[21] Hanratty and Walsh believe the problem is an engineering issue driven by 'market forces', which have demanded thinner, more flexible stents, but at the expense of longitudinal strength.[22]

There's a tragic irony in what shrinking stents can lead to: blocked arteries.

Earlier US government-sponsored evidence led to warnings of the limitations of stents, but these have been largely ignored by doctors, some of whom may view stents and angioplasty as a money-making, insurance-sponsored part of their practice.

Although, in the UK, only private doctors are likely to enjoy financial benefits like those of their American counterparts, the rationale for the increased use of stents has inevitably travelled across the Atlantic.

Benefits uncertain

A hospital survey carried out by a cardiology team at St Luke's Mid-America Heart Institute in Kansas City, Missouri, checked the statistics from more than 1,000 American hospitals across the country against guidelines developed by several medical organizations in 2009 for the appropriate use of stents. In the 71 per cent of cases that were true emergencies – the patient, for example, was having a heart attack – the team found that hospitals did a good job; 99 per cent of those procedures were deemed appropriate, although the researchers had to exclude 100,000 cases for lack of data.

Of the non-emergency remainder, the thousands of stents inserted as a just-in-case procedure for chronic but stable chest pain, 38 per cent – or 55,000 cases – were of uncertain benefit and a further 16,838 (12 per cent) were clearly inappropriate.[23] And in more than half of these inappropriate cases, the patient showed no evidence of heart disease whatsoever.

If these figures are extrapolated across the USA, then of the 700,000 patients receiving stents every year, 84,000 could be receiving them inappropriately – and many of these procedures will hasten a heart attack. Many doctors also believe these figures may be wildly conservative.

In 2007, the US Congress appropriated $1.1 billion (£724 million) to fund studies to determine which medical treatments deliver the best solutions at the most competitive cost. This is a rarity in the world of medicine, where health insurers – and indeed politicians – almost never call for studies into the most cost-effective medical procedures.

One such study, called COURAGE (Clinical Outcomes Utilizing Revascularization and Aggressive Drug Evaluation), rocked the world of cardiology when it was revealed that the 2,287 patients tracked for five years enjoyed no benefits in terms of preventing heart attack, stroke or death with either angioplasty or stents compared with a cocktail of generic heart drugs such as aspirin, beta blockers, calcium-channel blockers, blood vessel dilators and ACE inhibitors plus statins.[24]

Indeed, the day the news broke, shares of the leading stent maker Boston Scientific Corporation plummeted and, a month later, the number of stent implant procedures carried out in the USA fell by 13 per cent. Nevertheless, as soon as the headlines faded, the use of stents across the country quickly crept up to pre-COURAGE levels and has now peaked at some one million procedures per year.

Stents: a lucrative business

The reason doctors continue to use stents isn't difficult to find – if you follow the money. Each stent costs, on average, about $15,000 (£10,000) to implant and, every year in the USA alone, $15 billion (£10 billion) are spent on stent procedures.

What's more, a cardiologist receives about $900 (£600) per procedure – about nine times what he gets for a simple office visit for a heart drug prescription – and a hospital receives $10,000 (£6,500) per procedure.

Over the past decade, with improvements in stent design leading to an explosion in their deployment, US cardiologists installing stents made, on average, $500,000 (according to 2008 figures; or £280,000) – an increase of 22 per cent over the previous 10 years.

After publication of the COURAGE study, a Washington State agency called the Health Technology Assessment Program (HTAP) was considering putting the COURAGE research into practice and so commissioned a thorough review of the evidence that had supported the use of stents. However, at this point, a number of cardiologists joined together to fight the review and discredit the COURAGE findings.

When HTAP convened a conference call with representatives of stent-makers and cardiologists to request assistance in comparing stent and drug use, the industry and doctors declined to help.

As Mitchell Sugarman, senior director of health economics for stent maker Medtronic Inc., announced on the call, 'We don't want to end up being our own willing executioners.'

Atherectomy

This technique for unclogging heart vessels uses a thin flexible tube (catheter) with a sharp blade at the end to scrape away fatty deposits (plaques) from the inside of blood vessels. Claimed to be minimally invasive, it's meant to be an improvement over angioplasty by solving the thorny problem of restenosis. Yet, so far, it has performed poorly. In a study of 1,012 patients, the heart vessels of those undergoing atherectomy were indeed less blocked after treatment than those having angioplasty, but this apparent success was undermined by the fact that the probability of death or heart attack within six months was higher in the atherectomy group (8.6 per cent *vs* 4.6 per cent).[25] More recently, the COBRA (Comparison of Balloon Angioplasty versus Rotational Atherectomy) study, like earlier comparisons, found no differences between the two techniques in terms of deaths, symptom relief and restenosis.[26]

What to do instead

Perversely, those with heart disease who refuse the bypass, and opt simply to take drugs, or make dietary and lifestyle changes, can fare just as well, if not better, than those who have undergone the trauma of a procedure that involves cutting open the ribcage and stopping the heart for several hours.

Patients with angina or heart attack managed invasively with angioplasty or revascularization have twice the risk of a heart attack as those managed conservatively, and a 70 per cent greater risk of bleeding than those simply given drugs, according to a five-study review.[27] In fact, several studies show that the chances of survival following a mild heart attack are higher if the hospital doesn't immediately operate, but adopts a conservative approach instead. In a study by the US Veterans' Administration, more than three times as many bypass patients died compared with patients who were managed through 'watchful waiting'.[28] But bear in mind that 'doing nothing', as you might think of it, doesn't mean tucking into burgers and fries. It still requires a radical change in lifestyle, especially diet, and in any other factors that most probably brought on your heart disease in the first place.

Moreover, despite the impression given by many doctors, heart surgery is often not urgent. Dr Wayne Perry, a proponent of chelation therapy as an alternative to surgery (*see page 165*), suggests that patients should discuss with their doctor the possibility of deferring a heart operation for a year while they try other, less invasive methods of treatment, including stress management programmes combined with chelation therapy. Only if these other methods don't work should you think about going ahead with surgery.

The self-healing heart

The best medicine may be to do nothing – at first. When left to its own devices, a heart with obstructions in the main vessels somehow has the exquisite intelligence to embark on its own attempts at cure.

In three-quarters of cases, the heart will engineer the growth of new blood vessels to form its own natural bypass of the blocked arteries. These 'collaterals' keep blood flowing to the heart when the main vessels aren't working properly. Within three to six months, patients who do nothing at all may very well experience relief of their chest pain as a result of these new vessels.

However, collateral vessels tend to grow only when arterial narrowing and blockages arise slowly over time, as during the slow process of laying down plaques. When a vessel is suddenly blocked completely, such as by a blood clot, this is likely to cause a heart attack, an event the body can't prevent.

Collateral vessels vanish in bypass-surgery patients, and if the bypass doesn't take, the patient is then left in more danger than if they'd just kept their temporary 'detour' vessels intact.

Patients with a form of unstable or irregular angina are often lumped together as having 'acute coronary syndrome'. But it's been found that these patients don't benefit from early invasive interventions like angioplasty. This suggests that the self-healing mechanism of the heart may be disrupted in some way if doctors rush in too quickly to treat these patients.

|||||||||||||||||||||||||||||||||||||||||||

Part III

ALTERNATIVE SOLUTIONS

Chapter 9

THE BEST HEART-HEALTHY DIET

Conventional medicine is largely built upon the idea that any damage done to the body, especially the heart and its arteries, can't be undone when we're adults, and that symptoms can only be managed by drugs such as statins and antihypertensive agents until surgery becomes necessary. This dismal view boosts drug company revenues, as the vast majority of their income comes from drugs that manage chronic and intractable health problems such as cardiovascular disease. We might have been the architect of our own fate through poor diet, lack of exercise and smoking, but we can't also be the dismantler of the edifice of ill health that we've created for ourselves.

This belief, which sustains the pharmaceutical industry, has been confounded by two important studies that have a simple take-home message: it's never too late to heal yourself, particularly of heart disease. The small print is almost as heartening: the body is a dynamic, self-healing system.

Researchers from Northwestern University Feinberg School of Medicine in Chicago, Illinois, have concluded that anyone of any age who adopts the following five healthy lifestyle choices can control – and perhaps even reverse – their heart disease:

1. Keep a healthy body weight

2. Don't smoke

3. Engage in at least 30 minutes of moderate to vigorous physical activity five times a week

4. Don't drink more than one alcoholic drink a day if you're a woman, or more than two if you're a man

5. Eat a healthy diet, with lots of fresh fruit and vegetables.

Adopting all five points and sticking with them for 20 years or more can control and even reverse the symptoms of coronary artery disease such as calcification and thickening of the arteries. Each one of the five lifestyle changes reduces the chances of developing cardiovascular disease. On the other hand, people who take up unhealthy habits or lifestyles, such as becoming obese or a smoker, will see their odds of having heart disease increase.[1]

The Northwestern researchers assessed the impact of the five healthy lifestyle choices listed above in 3,538 young adults aged 18 to 30 who, despite their relative youth, were already showing signs of heart disease and atherosclerosis (arterial plaques). Their symptoms were only starting to appear, but didn't yet require drugs or other medical intervention.

After being monitored for 20 years, the cardio health of 25 per cent of these people had improved, while the 40 per cent who'd abandoned one or more of the options saw their condition worsen.

These findings debunk two of medicine's myths, says lead researcher Bonnie Spring. 'The first myth is that it's nearly impossible to change patients' behaviour. Yet we found that 25 per cent of adults made healthy lifestyle changes on their own. The second myth is that the damage has been done – adulthood is too late for healthy lifestyle changes to reduce the risk of developing coronary artery disease. Clearly, that's incorrect. Adulthood is not too late for healthy behaviour changes to help the heart.' Conversely, it would appear, adulthood is not the time to start unhealthy habits either.

The bottom line is that it's never too late. 'You're not doomed,' says Spring, 'if you've hit young adulthood and acquired some bad habits. You can still make a change and it will have a benefit for your heart.'

It's never too late

Even if you're in your 60s and adopt just one of the above five healthy options – say, losing some weight – you'll see a big improvement in the health of your heart and arteries.

To demonstrate the point, researchers from University College London (UCL) followed the health and wellbeing of 5,362 people all born in the same week in March 1946 in the UK. In 2010 at age 64, the UCL researchers chose 1,273 of them, and compared their weight and body fat to their risk profile for heart disease and atherosclerosis. As expected, those who were overweight or obese already had signs of atherosclerosis and high blood pressure, as well as diabetes. But the surprise was that those who modified their diet and lifestyle and dropped into a lower body mass index (BMI) category – from obese to overweight, or from overweight to normal weight – saw their risk of atherosclerosis and heart disease fall as well. And here's the really good news: losing weight for any length of time has long-term benefits, even if you put it back on again later.[2]

The Mediterranean approach

Many of the elements of what's now regarded as a healthy diet – simply prepared meat and fish, large helpings of fruits, vegetables, olive oil, nuts and fish – are part of the Mediterranean diet, commonly eaten in many southern European countries. A great deal of research now confirms that this sort of diet can help prevent heart attacks and even death. One astounding example of this was the Lyon Diet Heart Study, a prevention trial comparing the Mediterranean diet as followed in Crete with the 'prudent diet' usually prescribed for cardiac patients. After more than two years, all cardiovascular events, new heart attacks and deaths had decreased by 70 per cent among those eating the Mediterranean diet.[3]

This diet, followed by heart patients with no other interventions, yielded results more than twice as good as the very best results achieved by cholesterol-lowering drugs. When the researchers attempted to establish why, they found that the protective effects had nothing to do with blood cholesterol levels (whether the good or bad type). Instead, there were differences in levels of essential fatty acids (EFAs). The diet had higher intakes of *linolenic* and *oleic* acids (both of which are omega-3 fatty acids from fish and flaxseed oils) and lower intakes of saturated fats and *linoleic* acid (omega-6 fatty acids from corn, safflower and soya bean oils). This increase in linolenic and oleic acid, plus the decrease in linoleic acid, proved protective.

More recent evidence shows that the Mediterranean diet, including extra virgin olive oil and often nuts, reduces heart risk by 30 per cent.[4] And even if you have a family history of high cholesterol and stroke, you can reduce your risk by sticking to this diet, say researchers in Spain.[5]

What's the secret behind the Mediterranean diet? Researchers from the USA and UK think they've finally figured it out: it's the interplay between olive oil and leafy vegetables. When the unsaturated fats in olive oil come into contact with the nitrites in vegetables and salad greens, they form nitro fatty acids, which lower blood pressure – at least in the animal studies done so far.[6] Nuts and avocado may also do the job of olive oil.

A rich intake of antioxidants may also account for the protective effect of the diet. Higher levels of vitamins C and E were recorded with the Mediterranean diet, which is consistent with other studies showing that high levels of vitamin E and beta-carotene lower the risk of heart attack. It's generally accepted that Japanese and Mediterranean populations suffer far fewer heart problems than American and northern European populations, with mortality rates of 4–5 per cent and 12–15 per cent in these populations respectively. Vitamin A and beta-carotene levels are also higher in the Mediterranean diet, and intake of antioxidant-rich flavonoids is twice as high in Japan and the Mediterranean countries as in the USA and northern Europe.

When UK researchers studied nearly 11,000 health-conscious Brits, including vegetarians and people who frequently ate wholemeal bread, bran cereals, nuts, dried fruit, fresh fruit and raw salads, and compared their mortality levels with the rest of the population, after tracking them for nearly 17 years, they found that they were half as likely to suffer from heart disease or stroke as the rest of the population. Among these healthy eaters, those who ate fresh fruit every day had a 24 per cent reduction in fatal heart disease, a 32 per cent reduction in death from stroke and an overall 21 per cent lower death rate. The vegetarians had a 15 per cent lower rate of fatal heart disease, those who ate wholemeal bread every day had a 12 per cent lower death rate than the national average, while those who ate a raw salad every day had a 26 per cent lower rate of fatal heart disease.[7]

So simply increasing your intake of fruit and vegetables can dramatically lower your blood pressure,[8] probably because they're good sources of blood pressure-lowering potassium and fibre.[9]

Hypertensive people who increase their dietary fibre from fruit and veg, and their protein intakes, achieve an even more impressive fall in blood pressure. Those following a diet with protein intakes making up 25 per cent of total daily energy and a fibre intake of 27g every day saw, after eight weeks, a fall in 24-hour systolic blood pressure of 5.9mmHg.[10]

What's less well known is the role of potassium in blood pressure control. As it seems that people with higher dietary intakes of potassium have a lower incidence of stroke,[11] researchers at the University of Poona in India investigated whether potassium supplements, alone or with magnesium, benefited patients with mild hypertension. While blood pressure (and cholesterol) fell dramatically with additional potassium, adding magnesium offered no additional benefit.[12]

Several epidemiological surveys (that is, studies of diet in particular populations) have also suggested that people with low dietary levels of potassium are more likely to have hypertension – which explains why vegetarians, whose diets are often rich in potassium, have a lower incidence of the condition than the general population. As much of the potassium in vegetables is lost in cooking water if they are boiled for long periods of time, it's a good idea to steam or only lightly cook vegetables, and to regularly eat raw potassium-rich foods such as bananas.

Going raw is even more protective. Two or three servings a day of fruit, high in vitamin C and soluble fibre, can reduce the risk of heart disease by as much as 25 per cent.[13]

A low-glycaemic diet

Whole foods low in processed carbohydrates are another natural component of the Mediterranean diet. A more specifically low-carb diet was first developed in 1850 by William Banting in the first ever diet book and has, more recently, been popularized by the late French scientist Dr Michel Montignac. After using a low-carb/low-sugar diet to tackle his own diabetes, he discovered a sound explanation for why so many people fail with a low-fat or low-calorie diet. The problem with diabetes – and weight in general – isn't overeating, but overwhelming the pancreas for years with the secret sugars in bread, potatoes and, more especially, processed foods, causing the organ eventually to break down.

He concluded that overweight was the overnight motel on the long road towards having your pancreas and arteries pack up. Montignac's theory was simple: eat all you like of the foods that don't overtax insulin production by the pancreas and, eventually, the organ will heal and your body will return to its normal weight – as will your cholesterol.

However, Montignac's most important discovery wasn't just about weight loss or even diabetes, but perhaps one of the keys to understanding degenerative diseases. When patients remove hidden sugars from their diets, their cholesterol normalizes and their heart disease is reversed. Banting himself, who was growing deaf before he started the diet, got his hearing back after following it for a year.

The key to the Montignac diet is the glycaemic index (GI), a scoring system of a food's ability to raise blood sugar. Some carbs cause weight gain, while others can be eaten in large quantities with no worries. David Ludwig at the Children's Hospital in Boston, Massachusetts, says that every doctor should advise his patients to adopt the GI diet, specifically as a lifestyle choice to prevent diabetes, heart disease and obesity.

The diet differentiates between 'good' and 'bad' carbohydrates. Instead of banning all of them (like the Atkins and other high-fat diets), it instead rules out only those that rapidly increase blood glucose. This includes processed foods such as breakfast cereals, white bread, white rice, cakes, biscuits and, perhaps surprisingly, potatoes (especially fried) and drinks such as beer.

There's evidence that a low-carb diet can significantly reduce inflammation after six months, researchers at Linköping University in Sweden found.[14]

Low-GI foods include fruit, vegetables, pulses and grains (such as brown rice) that have not been overly processed. Meat is allowed, although Montignac recommended lean meat and lots of fish.

The glycaemic index (GI)

The GI measures the increase in blood sugar after eating a carbohydrate in relation to the effect of pure sugar (which scores 100). Sweetcorn has a score of 55, which means that it raises blood glucose by 55 per cent, or just over half as much as pure sugar does. In general, carbs below 55 are considered low GI, scores of 55–70 are mid-GI and those over 70 are high GI.

In the past, it was widely believed that simple sugars dramatically raise blood-glucose levels, while starches such as potatoes and bread are digested more slowly. The results of numerous studies show this is not so. One of the biggest surprises is potatoes, reported to have an average GI of 84, making them one of the higher GI foods around.

Initially, nutritionists analyzed foods by the amount of energy (calories) they provided. This was rather crudely worked out in a laboratory by burning foods to measure the amount of heat energy they produced. But caloric measures are useless for diabetics, who need to know the glucose value of foods to control their blood-glucose intakes and avoid the need for insulin injections. And the glucose values of foods can't be measured in the lab, but must be tested in living individuals.

This led to a painstaking series of tests in the 1980s, whereby every foodstuff was analyzed for its potential to produce glucose in the bloodstream. Human guinea pigs were fasted to create a baseline to measure against, then given a single food to eat. Regular blood samples were taken over four hours to chart changes in blood-glucose levels.

The results weren't quite as expected. One surprise was finding that all carbs caused a glucose peak roughly 30 minutes after ingestion. Previously, it had been thought that only simple carbs (like sugar and honey) were fast-acting, while complex ones (like potatoes and cereals) were slow-acting. There were dramatic differences in levels of blood glucose and, as the technical term for blood glucose is 'glycaemia', these differences were measured in terms of their glycaemic index: the higher the glucose peak, the greater the amount of blood glucose produced by that food.

Not surprisingly, virtually all foods have a GI lower than pure glucose. Also, as expected, the most refined carbohydrates led to the highest blood glucose levels. But there were unexpected findings too. Cooking was found to have major effects on the GI. Carrots, for example, produce three times the amount of blood glucose when cooked than when eaten raw. In fact, any cooking or processing raises the GI significantly.

'Bad' carbohydrates produce a sharp rise in blood glucose, causing hyperglycaemia, an excess of glucose in the bloodstream. These include all forms of white sugar (in processed snacks, sweets, biscuits and cakes), foods made from white flour such as bread and some pastas, and white rice. The Montignac diet also excludes all potatoes other than sweet potatoes and yams, as well as corn and beer.

'Good' carbohydrates cause only a slight increase in blood glucose. These include whole grains, brown rice, pulses such as lentils and dried beans, most fruits (ideally eaten on an empty stomach) and most vegetables high in fibre, such as leeks, cabbage, broccoli, cauliflower, salads and green beans.

Other foods that are relatively low GI are dried white pasta, barley, bulgur wheat, and wholegrain breads such as pumpernickel and rye. Incorporating these foods into the diet is associated with lower blood glucose, insulin and lipid (fat) levels.[15]

While simple and complex carbs can both increase blood sugar levels, the rate at which glucose is released varies. Foods with the same amounts of total carbohydrate can have different GI scores. Yams, for example, have a higher glycaemic effect than carrots, and kidney beans increase blood sugar levels more than soya beans. And the glycaemic effect of foods can indicate, as many researchers have found, the potential risk of much more than just acute sugar spikes.

One study from Hammersmith Hospital in London found that high-GI foods decrease levels of HDL (high-density lipoprotein) cholesterol, the 'good' type that safeguards against heart disease, so people who follow a low-fat diet and compensate by eating white rice or baked potatoes, for example, could be doing double the damage to their HDL cholesterol levels.[16]

Other research shows that processed 'white' food and drink such as sodas have a high GI and put stress on the arteries for several hours afterwards. Over time, the arteries' elasticity is lessened, possibly leading to heart disease or even sudden death from heart attack.

Researchers at Tel Aviv University showed how high-GI foods affect arterial health when they gave different foods to four groups of volunteers. Participants were given cornflakes, sugar, bran flakes or water (the placebo control) – and only those who drank water had normal arteries afterwards. The rest had poor arterial function that lasted for several hours. Arterial stress was especially evident in those given cornflakes or sugar, both high-GI foods.[17]

As with the Atkins regime, Montignac advocated two phases to his diet: phase one is to achieve weight loss; and phase two is to maintain your new lower weight.

The Montignac diet

It's thought that the amount of insulin triggered by a food remains the same however much of it you eat, and this theory appears to be supported by Montignac's diet. With this diet, you don't count carbs or calories, and you can consume any quantity of foods with a GI score of 50 or less.

The first, weight-loss phase lasts from one to three months, or until you reach your ideal weight. At this time, you can eat as much as you like, with plenty of protein and fats, because you're eating a balanced and varied diet from three substantial meals a day plus a snack – so long as the only carbs you eat have a GI score of 0 to 35.

While seven or eight pounds (three or three and a half kilos) of weight may be lost in the early weeks, a more reasonable target in the weeks thereafter is two to three pounds (about one kilo) a week.

Montignac described the second, maintenance phase as 'a more tolerant phase … Certain foods are no longer excluded and, in fact, previously banned foods can now be periodically reintroduced. It can therefore be viewed as the correct management of such dietary lapses.'

At this time, you can drink a reasonable amount of wine – up to half a litre per day – and have chocolate, but only the dark semisweet variety that's at least 70 per cent cocoa. You can eat foods with a GI score of 0 to 50 and carry on doing so for the rest of your life, as they will help you maintain your weight.

Montignac's prescient views on the link between a low-GI diet and heart disease have been borne out by science. The prestigious Cochrane Collaboration has now put its seal of approval on the diet as the best way to lose weight, with the added bonus of regularizing cholesterol levels. The Collaboration assessed six randomized controlled trials (or RCTs, considered the 'gold standard' of trial evidence) comparing the Montignac diet with diets that included foods with a higher GI score. The findings confirmed that the low-GI diet outperformed the others, and was especially good for people with obesity as it allowed them to eat many normal foods without having to stick to a rigid, restrictive diet plan. Those who stuck with the diet also saw their body mass index (BMI) scores, and total and LDL cholesterol levels, fall dramatically.[18]

What's more, in a study of 146 people with high blood pressure, nearly half were able to stop or reduce their heart drug treatment after following a low-carb diet. In contrast, only 21 per cent of those taking a drug while not following the diet reported similar reductions.[19]

Another comparison of low-GI, high-fat diets by Stanford University Medical School discovered that even though the diet was rich in saturated fats, it led to no changes in blood cholesterol levels, demonstrating once more that a low-sugar diet, rather than a low-fat diet, is the most heart-protective.[20]

The glycaemic index score chart

Unlike counting calories, the GI index doesn't measure a quantity of food, but is rather a scoring system ranging down from 100 (for pure glucose sugar). This means that, for example, whether you eat two slices of bread or the whole loaf, the GI score remains the same. (Just note that GI scores may vary slightly according to the organization assessing the foods.) For maximum heart health, stick to foods with a GI index of 50 or less, which includes meat and fish, most vegetables (other than some root veg), many fruits, and most whole grains. Avoid refined carbs (products made from flour and grains that have been processed and stripped of some of their nutrients), which are always converted to sugar in the body.

GI score (from high to low)			
Glucose (sugar)	100	Muesli	66
Parsnips (cooked)	97	Melon	65
French baguette	95	Beetroot (cooked)	64
Honey	87	Raisins	64
Potatoes (baked)	85	Bananas	62
Potatoes (fried)	75	Pastry	59
White rice	72	Sucrose (sugar)	59
Watermelon	72	Basmati rice	58
Bagel	72	Sweetcorn	55
Potatoes (boiled, new)	70	Sweet potatoes	54
White bread	70	Potato crisps	54
Ryvita	69	Kiwi fruit	52
Pineapple	66	Peas	51
Brown rice	66	White spaghetti	50

GI score (from high to low)			
Porridge oats	49	Plum	39
Carrots	49	Pear	38
Baked beans	48	Butterbeans	36
Instant noodles	46	Chickpeas	36
Wholegrain wheat bread	46	Black-eyed peas	33
Grapes	46	Haricot beans	31
Orange juice	46	Kidney beans	29
Wholemeal spaghetti	42	Lentils	29
Wholegrain rye bread	41	Barley	26
Apple juice	40	Grapefruit	25
Orange	40	Cherries	25
Apple	39	Soya beans	15

Other heart-healthy options

Besides watching your GI levels, the following are the best dietary ways to look after your heart:

Eat organic whole foods and opt for locally grown, seasonal, organic produce

Pesticides have been implicated in many illnesses, including infertility, cancer, birth defects, skin irritations and impotence. Organically reared animals fed on grass (which is what they're meant to eat), not grains, and organic produce not only contain substantially more of the basic nutrients than intensively farmed varieties, but also have up to 10,000 secondary nutrients essential for human health. As organic bacon and sausages may still include nitrates (which are carcinogenic), purchase them from sources that guarantee nitrate-free products.

Cook from scratch

Avoid anything canned, fried, preserved or laden with chemicals, or processed, refined or in any way interfered with. Vary your diet as much as possible: most allergy specialists claim that allergies are more likely to develop if you repetitively eat the same foods over long periods of time. Cut down on your consumption of food from tins and plastic bottles, which can leach bisphenol A (BPA), and avoid water sold in plastic bottles, as they may contain phthalates, which can mimic oestrogen, wreaking havoc in the body.

Eat a 'power breakfast'

Those who consume a large proportion of their total caloric intake in the morning tend to eat significantly less the rest of the day, which helps to control or prevent obesity.[21] Plus skipping breakfast increases your chances of a heart attack, high blood pressure and diabetes, especially in men.[22]

Don't limit saturated fats in favour of 'low-fat' or hydrogenated foods

The supposedly 'good' fats – polyunsaturated fats from vegetable oils (corn, soy, safflower and the like) – may predispose people to cancer, whereas animal fats may be protective, preventing heart disease, osteoporosis and even cancer. Two large studies have shown that regularly consuming more saturated fats leads to less disease progression than a diet higher in polyunsaturated fats and carbs.[23] And always avoid trans fats – produced by 'hydrogenation', whereby hydrogen is added to liquid vegetable oil to make it stay solid at room temperature – as they're clearly linked to a greater risk of heart disease.[24]

Get your omega-3 to omega-6 ratio right

Avoid an unhealthy ratio of omega-3 to omega-6 essential fatty acids (EFAs), as these fats regulate the major bodily functions, and deficiencies are behind many degenerative diseases. The modern Western diet's usual ratio is around 1 to 15–16.7 in favour of omega-6 EFAs, mostly because of the presence of high levels of vegetable oils (such as safflower, sunflower and corn oils) in processed foods. This ratio is known to promote many diseases, including cardiovascular disease. In contrast, diets high in omega-3 EFAs have disease-suppressing effects. In fact, diets that include just four times as much omega-6 as omega-3 are associated with a 70 per cent decrease in deaths related to heart disease.[25] To approach that ideal 4:1 ratio, as a general rule increase your intake of fish and take daily supplements of fish oils and food-grade flaxseed (or linseed) oil, which is 60 per cent omega-3 fat, and avoid processed food whenever you can.

Eat more beans

Increasing consumption of well-cooked pulses is an important part of a diet to reduce the risk of heart disease, according to a US population-based survey of more than 9,000 men and women without heart disease, who participated in the follow-up to the First National Health and Nutrition Examination Survey (NHANES I). Legume consumption was estimated from three-month food-frequency questionnaires for an average of 19 years. Compared with those eating legumes less than once a week, people who ate pulses four or more times a week had significant decreases in cardiovascular and heart-disease risk.[26]

Drink coffee in moderation

Compared with drinking less than a cup of coffee a day, people who drink four or more cups a day have a 20 per cent lower risk of any heart rhythm disturbance (arrhythmia), and the higher the coffee consumption, the less likely the need to be hospitalized for arrhythmias. These findings, based on 130,054 men and women, are surprising, as there's no explanation for how caffeine – coffee's most active ingredient – is able to reduce the risk of arrhythmias. Also, coffee contains cafestol, known to increase LDL cholesterol, which would be expected to increase the chances of abnormal heart rhythms.[27] Nevertheless, these findings are consistent with a Swedish study showing that people who drink three to four cups of coffee a day have a 25 per cent lower risk of stroke compared with those drinking just one cup a day or none at all.[28]

Eat foods rich in vitamin E

These include nuts, seeds, and corn and olive oils, and vitamin E is arguably the single most important nutrient for determining whether we live a long and healthy life. In a study of 698 men and women aged over 65, those with low blood levels of vitamin E saw a decline in their physical capabilities over a three-year period compared with those with higher levels of vitamin E. In fact, this was the only vitamin to have a direct impact on their physical wellbeing. Levels of vitamin D, iron and B vitamins, including folate, made no difference to the loss of physical function. The researchers believe that vitamin E, an antioxidant, prevents damage to muscles, nerve cells and DNA.[29]

Drink green tea

Frequent green-tea drinkers have lower cholesterol levels, and those who drink more than 10 cups a day also gain some protection against liver complaints. Researchers from the Saitama Cancer Center Research Institute in Japan are so excited by their findings, based on the tea-drinking habits of 1,371 men, that they're now looking into tea as a cancer preventative. Although this is one of the first studies of its kind,[30] a Spanish study has also suggested that drinking up to seven cups of green tea a day is a good choice for preventing heart disease.[31]

Eat dark chocolate

If you've had a heart attack, a bar of chocolate is probably the last thing your doctor would recommend. Yet new evidence suggests that chocolate could save your life by reducing your risk of a future fatal heart attack. Swedish researchers in the Stockholm Heart Epidemiology Program (SHEEP) quizzed more than a thousand heart attack survivors on their chocolate consumption, then followed them for eight years to see how they fared. The researchers found that the more chocolate consumed, the lower the risk of death due to heart disease – even after taking into account other risk factors such as obesity, smoking and alcohol consumption. Those who regularly indulged in chocolate – defined as two or more times a week – were up to three times less likely to die of heart problems than those who avoided chocolate. And even eating chocolate less than once a month had a significant protective effect.[32]

These findings are intriguing, though not surprising. Recently, the evidence has been stacking up that chocolate – far from being unhealthy – is actually a functional food with heart-protective properties. But beware: not all chocolate is created equal. Although SHEEP didn't distinguish between types of chocolate, other research indicates that it's only the dark kind that's good for the heart.

In one study, dark – but not white – chocolate dramatically reduced blood pressure in 20 mildly hypertensive patients who ate either 100g (3½oz) of dark chocolate or 90g (3oz) of white chocolate every day for two weeks. Only the dark chocolate caused systolic blood pressure to plummet by an average of 11.9mmHg and diastolic blood pressure by 8.5mmHg, making chocolate as effective as many of the antihypertensive drugs currently on the market.[33]

When doctors at the University of Cologne in Germany ran a similar study, but with less chocolate (just 6.3g/day, amounting to 30 calories' worth), remarkably even this small amount of dark chocolate – but, again, not white chocolate – was able to reduce blood pressure by almost 3mmHg. Although small, such a decrease applied across a population 'would reduce the relative risk of stroke mortality by 8 per cent, of coronary artery disease mortality by 5 per cent, and of all-cause mortality by 4 per cent', the researchers estimated.[34] As well as lowering blood pressure, dark chocolate increases 'good' HDL cholesterol while lowering 'bad' LDL cholesterol,[35] and also reduces platelet clumping (blood-clot formation)[36] while improving arterial endothelial function, including the production of nitric oxide, a vasodilator that helps to keep blood vessels clear of obstructions.[37]

The key ingredients in cocoa are flavanols, natural plant antioxidants already well known for their heart-healthy effects.[38] The Kuna Indians of Panama, for example, regularly eat large amounts of cocoa and suffer from little hypertension and stroke, despite eating salty food.[39]

Choose your fish carefully

Most catches are now tainted with industrial waste and mercury, and this applies even to 'farmed' fish, which have also been fed inappropriately with grains. Avoid swordfish, tuna and other deep-water fish, as they are likely to contain more mercury than smaller fish from shallower waters. And rotate your protein sources between different kinds of fish, meat, pulses and vegetable sources to minimize your exposure to specific chemicals.

Dump homogenized or pasteurized low-fat dairy

People who eat lots of dairy have higher levels of circulating insulin – such as growth factor (IGF)-1, which has been linked to a higher risk of many different cancers.[40] A Danish study also found that high (IGF)-1 levels increase the risk of chronic heart failure and deaths from all causes.[41]

Drink a moderate level of red wine

Alcohol advice seems to vary as much as the kinds of drink on offer, and is all very confusing and contradictory. We're told that excessive drinking increases your risk of liver disease, heart failure and cancer. Yet one US study found that people who upped their daily alcohol intake from very low (less than a glass of wine a day) to moderate (one or two glasses a day) 'significantly' reduced their risk of dying from a heart attack. It's thought that this is because moderate drinking increases levels of HDL cholesterol, which reduces heart disease risk.[42]

In a study looking at the components of the Mediterranean diet on their own, 'moderate ethanol consumption' (preferably wine) contributed 24 per cent to the low mortality rate seen with the diet.[43] But better make it red wine, as that contains health-giving resveratrol, which helps to reduce inflammation.[44]

Consider fasting

A day-long fast, during which you drink only water for 24 hours, lowers your chances of coronary artery disease and diabetes.[45] Fasting raises levels of adiponectin,[46] a protein that protects cardiovascular health by dilating blood vessels, and lowering inflammation and oxidative stress in both heart and blood vessel cells.[47]

What's the optimum dosage of EFAs you should be taking?

⇨ Attempt a ratio of 1:1 omega-6 to omega-3 fatty acids if you can, but the amount you take depends on your state of health and where you live. You probably don't need as much omega-3 if you live where it's sunny and warm most of the time.

⇨ If you're ill, nutritionists recommend 300mg of EPA and DHA (*see page 45*) for every 10lb (4.5kg) of body weight. This equates to 1tbsp (15ml) of an average cod liver oil, or 10 capsules, for a 130lb (59kg) person.

⇨ Use olive oil, coconut oil or butter instead of other plant oils for cooking.

⇨ Take EFAs with other supplements. As they are fragile and easily oxidized, leading to harmful free radicals, always take them in a supplement using naturally derived vitamin E.

⇨ EFAs require other nutrients to be converted in the body. Ensure that you're taking adequate amounts of vitamins B and C, as well as magnesium, calcium and zinc.

⇨ Ensure that your brand of fish oil is free of mercury and PCBs (polychlorinated biphenyls). This will require some detective work such as contacting the manufacturer and examining independent reports of the product.

⇨ Buy products containing a therapeutic dose of vitamin E, which will prevent the oil from going rancid.

⇨ If you're vegetarian, you can take flaxseed or walnut oil as your omega-3. However, you should be aware that both oils contain the precursor alpha-linolenic acid (ALA), which needs to be converted to EPA and DHA for optimal benefit. This conversion process is not particularly efficient and grows worse with age (especially if you also have raised insulin levels, as these will inhibit delta-6-desaturase, the enzyme necessary to convert ALA to EPA and DHA).

Heart-healthy superfoods

Eat as many of these superfoods as you can, in main meals and as snacks:

⇨ **Nuts:** Eating walnuts three times a week can nearly halve your chances of dying from heart disease.[48] They raise levels of 'good' HDL cholesterol, and their oil helps to maintain strong blood vessels.[49] The same goes for pecans, which contain the antioxidant gamma-tocopherol, a form of vitamin E. Gamma-tocopherol lowers LDL cholesterol, improves arterial health and reduces inflammation.[50] And new evidence from Aston University in Birmingham shows that just snacking on 50g of almonds a day increases the amount of antioxidants in the bloodstream, reduces blood pressure and improves blood flow – again perhaps owing to vitamin E.[51]

⇨ **Apples and pears:** Eating just one apple or pear (the so-called 'white' fruit) every day nearly halves the risk of stroke, possibly because both are rich in quercetin, a flavonoid.[52] In fact, fruit (and vegetables) may be as effective as a statin in reducing cholesterol, but without the nasty side-effects.[53] Eating one apple a day (actually, the peel) may also protect against atherosclerosis, as shown by animal studies.[54]

⇨ **Raisins:** A handful of raisins three times a day has a dramatic effect, lowering systolic and diastolic blood pressure by up to 7 per cent, possibly owing to the potassium in the fruit.[55]

⇨ **Beetroot juice:** One 230fl oz (8fl oz) glass of beetroot juice a day can lower your blood pressure by around 10mmHg. Dark-green leafy vegetables or even a bowl of lettuce may have the same effect, as they are rich in nitrate/nitrite, part of the nitric oxide pathway that reduces blood pressure, inhibits blood clots and improves vascular function.[56]

⇨ **Pulses:** Just eating one serving (130g/4½oz, or about half a cup) of pulses such as beans, lentils or chickpeas every day can significantly lower so-called 'bad' LDL cholesterol levels.[57]

⇨ **Tomatoes:** These fruits contain lycopene, which seems to improve the health and function of blood vessels. In one study, lycopene supplements relaxed the blood vessels of heart patients by 53 per cent. The lycopene in tomatoes is even more potent when the fruit is cooked and puréed, as in ketchup.[58]

Your heart-healthy supplement programme

Unless you live on a farm, grow all your own organic vegetables and have access to free-range meat, it's almost certain you'll have vitamin deficiencies despite the best of diets – largely because food isn't as nutritious as it once was, owing to the way it's now slaughtered, picked, baked or processed, and the length of time it sits on supermarket shelves. Most of us don't get enough selenium, for example, and this deficiency alone can trigger a range of age-related diseases such as heart disease and cancer, say researchers from the Children's Hospital Oakland Research Institute in California.[59] Selenium can also protect against oxidative stress, which leads to tissue damage, and has particular effects on heart tissue and cardiovascular health in general.[60]

Even standard doses of vitamin D supplements can help us to live longer. Vitamins D2 (ergocalciferol) and D3 (cholecalciferol) have protective effects against life-threatening cardiovascular disease, say researchers.[61] Furthermore, taking multivitamins, including A, most of the B family, C, D and E, can cut the risk of heart attacks nearly by half, even when taken for five or more years with no other supplements. The protective effect is strongest in women with no history of heart disease.[62]

Ideally, before embarking on supplementation, you should get yourself tested by a knowledgeable nutritionist to determine which nutrients you need or aren't getting from your food, and customize your supplement programme accordingly. That said, here are the supplements virtually anyone with a heart problem could benefit from:

⇨ **Take a good-quality multivitamin/mineral supplement:** Choose a good multivitamin/mineral supplement made with natural products and few fillers and produced by a reputable manufacturer (and not a pharmaceutical company, which tends to produce cheap and mass-produced forms of vitamins).

⇨ **Make antioxidants the mainstay of your supplement programme:** Low levels of selenium can increase blood clot formation (platelet aggregation) and constrict blood vessels; on the other hand, an increase in selenium levels by 50 per cent is able to reduce heart disease risk by 24 per cent.[63] Two studies, by the Harvard School of Public Health and Channing Laboratory in Boston, Massachusetts, found that high intakes of vitamin E can lower the risk of coronary heart disease in men and women.[64] The vitamin also protects the heart when taken as pre-treatment before coronary bypass surgery.[65]

Furthermore, the lower your blood levels of vitamin A and beta-carotene (as well as other antioxidants such as vitamins C and E), the higher your risk of angina, so make sure you're getting enough.[66]

Suggested daily dosages: up to 25,000IU (international unit) as beta-carotene or 10,000IU as retinol, a form of vitamin A derived from animals, 1–3g of vitamin E or up to 600IU as tocotrienols, 10–50mg of zinc and up to 200mcg of selenium.

Note: Don't take higher levels of vitamin E except under the close supervision of a qualified health practitioner.

⇨ **Vitamin C:** Even a marginal vitamin C deficiency can contribute to cardiovascular diseases such as atherosclerosis and angina.[67] This vitamin reduces blood levels of high-sensitivity C-reactive protein (hsCRP), a marker of inflammation and an important cause of cardiovascular disease. Heart patients are twice as likely to die within a year if their vitamin C levels are low, whereas just eating your five-a-day portions of fruit and veg will provide enough vitamin C to reduce your risk of fatal heart failure by more than two times.[68] Nevertheless, to be on the safe side, do take a supplement as well.

Suggested daily dosage: 1–3g or more (with the guidance of a trained nutritional therapist)

⇨ **B vitamins:** If you've had a heart attack or heart disease, high levels of B6 protect your heart against further damage, and thiamine (B1) can improve your heart's pumping function,[69] while niacin, or nicotinic acid (B3), can increase HDL ('good') cholesterol. Ignore the recent bad press about niacin, which only happened because the vitamin was paired with Merck's new lipid-lowering drug laropiprant (Tredaptive in Europe and Cordaptive in the USA). Patients developed muscle weakness, a known side-effect of statins.[70] Not surprisingly, this drug combination was recalled in January 2013.

According to Steven Nissen, past president of the American College of Cardiology, 'Niacin is really it. Nothing else available is that effective.' Nissen's opinion is seconded by Mayo Clinic researcher William Parsons, who says it 'decreases the incidence of coronary disease and strokes, and raises life expectancy'.[71]

Suggested daily dosages: 100mg of vitamin B6, 50mg of thiamine; get your body used to niacin by starting with a 25mg dose with food (easily done by chopping a 100mg tablet into four pieces) and, after a few days, increasing the dose to 50mg, then increasing it again after a few more days. The optimal therapeutic dose is 400mg.

⇨ **L-carnitine:** Made in the body from amino acids (lysine and methionine), high doses of this compound delivered intravenously reduce ventricular arrhythmias after a heart attack.[72] An Italian review also found that patients taking this supplement enjoyed a reduction in the incidence of death and heart failure after leaving the hospital; in another study of 537 patients with heart failure, l-carnitine improved their exercise capacity and preserved their heart function.[73]

Suggested daily dosage: 250–750mg

⇨ **Coenzyme Q10:** CoQ10 can prevent heartbeat irregularities and the cell and tissue damage usually seen after a heart attack.[74] Choose a formula that contains ubiquinol, which is more readily taken up for use by the body.[75]

Suggested daily dosage: 60–100mg (or higher with supervision)

⇨ **Omega-3 fatty acids:** As noted earlier (*see page 44*), these are known to be heart-protective, as they markedly reduce 'bad' cholesterol and triglycerides while increasing 'good' HDL.[76] But if you're taking these fatty acids as supplements, make sure you also increase your intake of vitamin E to prevent possible cellular damage.

Suggested daily dosage: 1,000–1,500mg as fish oil

⇨ **Chromium and magnesium:** According to a large-scale study by the renowned British laboratory-testing service, Biolab Medical Unit, which is based in central London, people become deficient in both chromium and magnesium with age, and both are necessary for heart health. Magnesium is essential for bone health and more absorbable than calcium supplements, and lowers blood pressure too.[77]

Suggested daily dosage: 100mcg of chromium, 200–600mg of magnesium

⇨ **Vitamin D:** About a third of the general population is vitamin D-deficient. Yet this vitamin offers natural protection against most types of heart disease, while boosting vascular function and immunity too. People who regularly supplement with vitamin D increase their longevity by 7 per cent. The body naturally produces it from sunlight – just five to 15 minutes of sun per day between 10 a.m. and 3 p.m., without sunscreen, should do the job.[78] If you sunburn easily, make sure you avoid the hottest midday sun and take natural sunscreen supplements (*see page 186*).

Suggested daily dosage: 600–1,000IU vitamin D, 400–1,000IU if age 18 or under

⇨ **'Good guy' bacteria:** Invest in a high-quality probiotic that includes lactobacilli, bifidobacteria, S*accharomyces boulardii*, non-disease-causing strains of *Escherichia coli* and streptococci, as it's suggested in a review of nine studies that the more bacterial species in the mix, the better. The same review also found that such a supplement can lower blood pressure, but be patient: it may take at least eight weeks before you see any results.[79]

Chapter 10

PROVEN ALTERNATIVE TREATMENTS FOR HEART DISEASE

In the view of standard medicine, heart disease – its deadliest and most intractable adversary – can only be vanquished by the most powerful drugs, the most sophisticated surgery and the most advanced state-of-the-art technology. Ask most doctors about non-drug approaches and they'll reply that attempting to treat this disease with alternative medicine is like trying to cure cancer with a facial.

But this view ignores the clear scientific evidence that many alternative approaches are far more potent against heart disease than all of medicine's weapons put together. However, the alternative method is not a matter of finding that one magic bullet that will erase all your symptoms. Effective care for patients with heart disease depends on how well doctors understand the whole patient. Tackling heart disease holistically requires a four-pronged approach: cleaning up your diet (see Chapters 1, 4 and 9); having a regular exercise regime (see Chapter 11); making use of a number of holistic options and supplements (Chapter 9); and creating a highly supportive social network (Chapter 12).

This chapter examines those alternative treatments showing evidence of success for a variety of heart conditions.

Lowering your blood pressure naturally

One good way to begin repairing your heart is by reducing your blood pressure, which can be a warning sign for stroke, heart attack and heart failure, aneurysms (blood clots in the brain), peripheral artery disease and even chronic kidney problems.

But even if your blood pressure is over the so-called 'normal' 140/90mmHg and you're terrified that your high blood pressure will lead to a heart attack or stroke, some simple lifestyle changes can usually bring your blood pressure back to normal. You can try these suggestions one at a time or several together, although it's best to work with a healthcare practitioner experienced in non-drug methods of blood pressure control. The following tried-and-tested naturopathic tips are from *What Doctors Don't Tell You*'s resident naturopath and 'medical detective', Dr Harald Gaier:

⇨ **Lose weight:** There's no question that weight affects your blood pressure[1] and that losing pounds, if you're significantly overweight, lowers it.[2] But ignore the body mass index (BMI), a clumsy and imprecise measure of obesity and the main method used to assess ideal weight. It's arrived at through a complicated computation, which involves dividing your weight by your height, and the result is a number. If you're slightly over the 'ideal' number for your weight and height, you're overweight; if you're way over, you're obese. Nevertheless, when researchers recently analyzed 40 studies that involved more than 250,000 people, they found that obese people, as defined by the BMI, had far fewer cardiovascular problems or were living longer than their leaner counterparts. Only the people who were underweight or seriously obese, according to the BMI measure, were more likely to suffer a heart condition. The problem, according to the researchers, is the BMI measure itself, which doesn't differentiate between fat and lean mass, and so fit people with muscles are classified as overweight according to the BMI.[3] Instead of the BMI, use common sense to determine if you're seriously overweight.

⇨ **Avoid processed carbs:** A low glycaemic index (GI) diet can regularize your metabolism, help you lose weight, reduce blood sugar and insulin levels, and lower blood pressure[4] (*see page 137*).

⇨ **Organic apple cider or wine vinegar:** Taken daily, this works like an ACE inhibitor by inhibiting the renin-angiotensin hormones that regulate blood pressure balance. When too much angiotensin is secreted owing to an overactive hormone system, blood vessels constrict.[5]

Suggested daily dosage: 15ml (1tbsp) in half a glass of water

⇨ **Watermelon (*Cucurbita citrullus*) extract:** This can dilate capillaries, the tiny blood vessels that run between arteries and veins. In one study, l-citrulline supplements significantly reduced the risk of a serious cardiac event in obese adults with high blood pressure.[6]

Suggested daily dosage: 2–3g of l–citrulline (available online)

⇨ **Garlic:** A review of 11 studies found that garlic preparations significantly reduced high blood pressure.[7]

Suggested daily dosage: 600–900mg of garlic powder

⇨ ***Achillea wilhelmsii* extract:** This Iranian plant (a member of the Asteraceae family) significantly lowered blood pressure after six months.[8]

Suggested daily dosage: 15–20 drops twice daily of a liquid extract made up of water with a little alcohol as a preservative

⇨ **Tomato extract:** Patients given 250mg/day of Lyc-O-Mato gel capsules, containing 15mg of lycopene plus other carotenoids, enjoyed significant reductions in blood pressure after just two months.[9]

⇨ **Bioactive peptides:** These naturally occurring peptides (chains of amino acids) are derived from plants and animals, and act like ACE inhibitor drugs to lower blood pressure.[10] Again, these are available online.

⇨ **Homeopathic Cytisus Laburnum:** Prepared from the flowers and young leaves of wild laburnum, this remedy has worked for many patients. It has also been put through a modern homeopathic proving to test its effects.[11] Proving trials involve giving the tested homeopathic remedy to healthy individuals and analyzing the symptoms that arise; if the same symptoms arise in healthy people as those the remedy is meant to treat in people who are ill, the remedy is viewed as having a 'proving'.

Suggested daily dosage: 6DH potency twice daily

⇨ **Aged garlic extract:** This can lower blood pressure in patients with high blood pressure, particularly if they haven't been helped by antihypertension drugs.[12]

⇨ **Magnesium supplements:** This all-purpose heart supplement reduces blood pressure by relaxing blood vessel walls.[13]

⇨ **Biofeedback:** Learn to unwind and control your own blood pressure with the StressEraser®, a portable biofeedback device that teaches you how to activate your own 'relaxation response', a physical state of deep rest that counteracts the negative effects of the stress response – the release of stress hormones like cortisol and adrenaline – by revealing your heart rate on a screen, which you then synchronize to your breathing. (The device is available online in the UK at www.stresseraser-uk.com.)

Treating atherosclerosis

Like blood pressure, furred-up arteries can also be successfully treated without resorting to drugs or surgical procedures. Here are the best alternative treatments:

Chelation therapy

Said to be a safer alternative to surgery and drugs for preventing atherosclerosis, this treatment uses molecules called 'chelators', which target stray atoms and chemically bind to them, so allowing metals to be excreted from the body.

Chelators have been licensed by the US Food and Drug Administration since the 1950s for toxic metal overload, especially lead, mercury and aluminium, and for nutritional metals such as copper and iron when they become stored in the wrong places in the body. One of the by-products of chelation is improvement in the function of arteries previously blocked by plaque. Some believe that heavy metal loads in the body as well as compounds like calcium are responsible for atherosclerosis. By removing metals and excess calcium from the body, chelation therapy removes the instigator of clogged arteries.

When chelation is used to treat heart disease, the patient is given intravenous infusions of disodium ethylenediaminetetraacetic acid (EDTA), along with vitamins C and B, electrolytes, procaine and heparin, to chemically 'grab' and remove the fatty deposits on arterial walls.

Chelation generally involves between 20 and 40 infusions of EDTA via a slow drip into the blood, usually given twice a week. As EDTA moves through the patient's bloodstream, it binds with artery-clogging deposits and then passes out of the body, taking the deposits with it. Many organizations in the UK and USA have enthusiastically taken up chelation therapy, including the Arterial Disease Clinic in London and Lancashire (UK), and the American College of Advancement in Medicine (ACAM). Lists of chelation clinics can be found on the internet.

After years of controversy, chelation was finally given a cautious thumbs-up by 329 collaborators with the Columbia University Division of Cardiology who were involved in a large-scale randomized controlled trial (the 'gold standard' for evidence) showing that it modestly reduced the chances of adverse events following a heart attack.[14]

However, a note of caution: earlier research found that chelation may cause kidney damage in patients with kidney disease if the treatment delivery doesn't strictly adhere to the proper protocol.[15] If you do wish to try chelation therapy, it's vital that you find a highly experienced doctor or clinic you can rely on to follow the ACAM protocol strictly.

It's also important that you follow the full programme for cardiovascular disease, including the optimal diet, appropriate nutritional supplements, regular exercise programme and stress management. The Arterial Disease Clinic in the UK will accept people in any condition, be they gangrene sufferers, stroke victims or bypass and angioplasty failures.

Chelation therapy can be expensive. The usual 40-infusion treatment may cost more than $5,000 (£3,300) in the USA, although some doctors offer an 'abbreviated' form for mild cases at a reduced rate. (While making your comparisons, bear in mind that the hospital charge for bypass surgery is, on average, $123,000/£81,000, including the doctor's fee.) If you're considering chelation therapy, Dr Wayne Perry of London's Wimpole Street advises:

⇨ Check that the doctor is experienced in chelation and will be following the ACAM protocol. (The drugs used are widely available, and there is nothing to stop any doctor from offering the treatment.)

⇨ Check that the doctor will be monitoring your kidney function before and after chelation.

⇨ Find out in advance exactly what drugs will be used, and do your own research to make sure you're happy about the proposed treatment.

In the UK, the best bet is to contact the Arterial Disease Clinic in London or in Lancashire (tel: 01942 676 617). In the USA, contact ACAM (380 Ice Center Lane, Suite C, Bozeman, Montana 59718; website: www.acam.org) or call 1 800 532 3688 to find a physician in your area.

Other alternative treatments for furred arteries

The following approaches have evidence of success:

⇨ **Meditation:** This ancient practice, valued by Eastern religions, of concentrated mind focus aims to slow down brain waves in waking consciousness to a preponderance of slower 'alpha' waves (8–13 cycles per second), promoting relaxation of the autonomic nervous system and heart rate. Meditation can help heart patients lower their risk of an inadequate blood supply to the heart (ischaemia) due to blood vessel narrowing and thereby lower the risk of a fatal heart attack.[16]

⇨ **Acupuncture:** This 5,000-year-old treatment, also from the East, rests on the theory that the body has fields of energy, or 'ch'i,' channelled through pathways called 'meridians'. Blockages of this energy cause diseases, but they can be successfully treated by inserting needles into certain points along the meridians, which re-establish the free flow of energy. Acupuncture has been subjected to some 10,000 scientific trials, much of the research validating its use for a number of conditions, particularly pain relief. With heart conditions, patients receiving acupuncture are able significantly and safely to increase the work capacity of their hearts.[17]

⇨ **Blue-green algae:** Also known as 'cyanobacteria', these primitive microorganisms have proved in numerous studies to prevent cardiovascular disease and non-alcoholic fatty liver disease, linked to type 2 diabetes, by lowering blood lipids, inflammation and oxidative stress. In fact, they can be said to be protective against a wide range of metabolic and inflammatory diseases such as diabetes and atherosclerosis.[18]

Plant-based remedies

A qualified, experienced herbalist may prescribe the following herbs, which can help clear your arteries when given in therapeutic dosages:

⇨ **Bromelain**, derived from pineapple, can ease angina and various cardiovascular disorders,[19] as can hawthorn extract (*Crataegus* species).[20]

⇨ **Ginger (*Zingiber officinale*)**, a recognized blood-thinner, can halt the development of atherosclerosis (fatty deposits in blood vessel walls) and ischaemic heart disease too.[21]

⇨ ***Ginkgo biloba*** can reduce pain in heart patients, help them walk over longer distances, and also 'thin' the blood of patients with arteriosclerotic disorders.[22]

⇨ ***Terminalia arjuna***, an Indian medicinal plant, can reduce the signs and symptoms of heart failure.[23]

⇨ **Chinese herbs**, a number of which can have profound effects on the heart. *Andrographis paniculata* Nees (also known in Indian Ayurvedic medicine as *Bhui-neem*), for example, has proved useful for preventing recurrent narrowing of arteries after angioplasty.[24]

⇨ **Gugulipid**, derived from the resin of the guggul tree (*Commiphora mukul*), is a lipid-lowering Ayurvedic remedy that can prevent atherosclerosis and raise 'good' HDL in 60 per cent of cases, while lowering 'bad' LDL cholesterol significantly.[25]

Easing angina

Angina offers a first-class example of the formidable self-healing power of the body. Contrary to popular belief, this sign of inadequate oxygen to the heart muscle won't inevitably lead to heart disease, but can instead often lower the risk of a heart attack and improve the patient's prognosis, owing to so-called 'preconditioning'.[26]

After a bout of (non-fatal) ischaemia (temporarily obstructed blood flow to the heart), the heart muscle receives a sudden renewal of blood supply, which can protect against heart attack by washing away any accumulations during the ischaemia. Also, those with long-term 'stable angina' develop connections between vessels (anastomoses) that allow what's known as 'collateral blood flow'.[27] Although medicine still doesn't understand preconditioning, studies suggest it may have something to do with an enzyme called 'protein kinase C'.[28]

Also, during angioplasty, when the balloon catheter is inflated within a coronary artery to stretch the vessel and push aside any obstructions, the balloon itself temporarily obstructs blood flow, leading to 'transient myocardial ischaemia' or reduced blood flow to the heart, rather like a sharp attack of angina. This means that angioplasty itself can prompt preconditioning and so ease angina.[29]

Alternatives that can help with angina

A wide variety of alternative remedies have shown evidence of success in easing the pain of angina:

⇨ **Homeopathy:** Tinctures of *Crataegus oxyacantha* (hawthorn) are widely and successfully used by homeopaths, and can protect the heart after ischaemic episodes.[30]

⇨ **Coenzyme Q10 (ubiquinone):** Patients with stable angina taking 150mg/day of this supplement in three doses experienced reductions in frequency of angina attacks and also in the need for nitroglycerin (the standard spray for emergency use by people at risk of a heart attack), and they were also able to increase the duration of their exercise significantly.[31] A pooled analysis of 13 studies of CoQ10 for congestive heart failure concluded that it can increase left ventricular output in such patients.[32]

⇨ **Herbs:** Extracts derived from *Ammi visnaga* (khella) fruit (called visnadin, khellin and visnagin) can act like calcium-channel blockers against angina.[33] Khella can improve blood flow to the heart and relax coronary blood vessels and, when used continuously, may even stop or reduce frequency and severity of angina attacks as well as the pain.[34]

⇨ **Barberry root bark:** Extracts of *Berberis vulgaris* bark can both treat and prevent ventricular fibrillation (seriously abnormal heart rhythms) caused by scarring from a previous heart attack or ischaemia.[35]

⇨ **Proteolytic enzymes:** These usually help to break down protein into amino acids. The enzyme bromelain, derived from the pineapple plant, can break down the fibrin in blood clots, making it particularly helpful for heart patients with angina and related cardiovascular disorders. In one study, angina patients taking 1,200mg/day of bromelain were entirely symptom-free three months later (with some as early as four days after starting treatment); their symptoms returned as soon as they stopped taking the enzyme.[36]

⇨ **Ayurvedic medicine:** Abana, an Ayurvedic combination containing *Terminalia arjuna*, *Withania somnifera*, *Tinospora cordifolia*, *Boerhaavia diffusa* and *Nardostachys jatamansi*, can significantly improve left ventricular output, and lower blood pressure by reducing the stress put on the heart as it expands and contracts to pump enough blood around the body.[37]

Talk, listen and pray

'Coronary heart disease is not just physical, but also has a psychological component,' says Dr Zoi Aggelopoulou, who has studied heart-attack survivors in her coronary care unit at the NIMTS Veterans Hospital in Athens, Greece. She noticed that her patients were less likely to suffer a second attack, die or return to hospital if doctors talked to them about their treatment, let them listen to music or helped religious patients say their prayers. While looking more deeply into the subject, she reviewed nine studies that assessed the benefits of psychological interventions on heart patients, and found that they supported her own observations: psychological interventions reduced the risk of death and a second heart attack by 55 per cent over a two-year period.[38]

Preventing stroke

To minimize your chances of suffering a stroke, take some of the following:

⇨ **B vitamins:** These reduce levels of homocysteine, an amino acid in the blood that's linked to stroke and heart disease.

Suggested daily dosage: 1mg folic acid or vitamin B9, 10mg B6, 400mcg B12

⇨ **Garlic:** This natural blood-thinner can dramatically lower the risk of blood clots in just four weeks.[39]

Suggested daily dosage: 800mg of garlic powder

⇨ *Gingko biloba:* Another powerful blood-thinner, this can reduce blood platelet build-up across all dosages.

Suggested daily dosage: 120–600mg

⇨ **Ginger:** After just one week of daily consumption, this powerful herb can lower blood-clotting agents in the circulation.

Suggested daily dosage: 5g (raw)

⇨ **Qigong:** This ancient Chinese form of exercise is particularly effective for reducing stroke risk. In one study, just 18 per cent of hypertensive patients who regularly practised qigong died of stroke compared with 41 per cent among those who didn't do this exercise.[40]

A final point that must be emphasized is: **don't smoke**. And even if you're a non-smoker, try to keep away from smoke-filled rooms, as even second-hand smoke can increase the likelihood of stroke.[41]

Recovering from stroke

If you've suffered a stroke, a number of alternative therapies can speed recovery:

⇨ **Music therapy:** Music can have powerful effects on the brain, and listening for a few hours a day can boost brain function, especially in the early stages following a stroke, according to a study from Finland. In one study, recovery of verbal memory and focused attention (the ability to control and perform mental operations, and resolve conflicts) improved significantly more in stroke victims who listened to music than in control groups who didn't. The music group also felt less depressed and confused than the non-music group. What's more, these differences were still evident six months later, suggesting that music may have long-term effects on brain function and mood.[42]

Another compelling study looked at the effects of music on three stroke patients who'd lost half their field of vision, a condition known as 'visual neglect'. The patients completed tasks under three conditions: listening to music they liked; listening to music they didn't like; and in silence. While listening to music of their liking, the patients showed greater responses in the parts of their brain related to emotion and attention, which eventually led to decreases in their visual neglect.[43]

⇨ **Guided imagery:** This technique, which involves visualizing a desired physical outcome, has helped people recover from stroke, especially in cases where mobility has been affected. In one study, 32 chronic stroke patients with limited arm movement were able to carry out more 'activities of daily living' after six weeks of 30-minute guided imagery sessions twice a week than those who did other therapeutic exercises.[44]

⇨ **Video games:** Virtual reality and other interactive 'videogaming' are new therapies being offered to people following a stroke. These involve computer-based programmes designed to simulate real-life objects and events. A review of 19 trials involving 565 participants found that arm function and the ability to deal with everyday activities were significantly improved in those who played the games.[45]

⇨ **Tai chi:** Exercise is good for stroke victims, and tai chi, the Chinese 'slo-mo' form, is especially beneficial. It can improve balance, lower blood pressure and improve mood too.[46]

⇨ **Vitamin B3 (niacin) therapy:** This may help to improve brain function after a stroke by rewiring the brain through stimulation of new blood vessel growth and new nerve cells – although so far this has only been demonstrated in lab rats.[47] In people, niacin raises HDL cholesterol and lowers the risk of cardiovascular events in those at high risk, suggesting that it may be an effective treatment for stroke patients with low blood HDL levels.[48]

Treating heart flutters (atrial fibrillation)

Although atrial fibrillation in itself isn't necessarily life-threatening, it can require emergency treatment (such as with a defibrillator) and may also lead to complications, such as stroke or heart failure. Conventional medicine usually tries to treat this disorder of the heart's electrical signalling with drugs or pacemakers, but *What Doctors Don't Tell You*'s resident naturopath Dr Harald Gaier has evidence that many types of alternative medicine can actually achieve everything that conventional treatments attempt.

⇨ **Herbs:** *Sarothamnus scoparius* (Scotch broom; also known as *Cytisus scoparius*) is an effective non-toxic herbal medicine long known to work for various cardiac and circulatory problems. It's particularly useful for resolving both atrial and ventricular fibrillation, and also acts as a diuretic, which helps to remove excess fluid and lower blood pressure.[49] The seeds and flowers can be used to make a weak infusion.

Suggested dosage for S. scoparius: 1tbsp (10ml) three or four times a day

The herb's medicinal effectiveness as a cardiac and circulatory therapy was solidly established nearly a century ago, and extracts of Scotch broom are available online in both the USA and UK. One licensed standardized extract called Spartiol® Cardiohom (made by Dr Gustav Klein GmbH & Co., Zell am Harmersbach, Germany) is approved by the German Medicinal Registration Authority, which monitors medicinal herbal preparations. This should not be self-prescribed, though; and if taken over the long term, its use must be monitored by the prescribing healthcare professional.

Suggested dosage for Spartiol Cardiohom: seven drops in half a glass of water three times a day

⇨ **Homeopathy:** The homeopathic version of Scotch broom has undergone a two-year proving trial.[50] According to George Vithoulkas, professor of homeopathic medicine, Spartium Scoparium 'increases the strength of the heart, slows it and reduces blood pressure'.[51]

Recommended potency: 2DH

Other remedies for fibrillation with demonstrated success are Hoitzia Coccinea and Hydrophis Cyanocinctus.[52]

Recommended potencies: 3DH for Hoitzia Coccinea, 4CH for Hydrophis Cyanocinctus

⇨ **Acupuncture:** This traditional Chinese medical technique can also work wonders for heart rhythm problems. In Dr Harald Gaier's experience, heart flutters can stop on the spot just by needling three acupoints: H5, or Tong Li; H7, or Shen Men; and H8, or Shao Fu.[53]

⇨ **Magnesium therapy:** An extensive review of 12 randomized controlled trials involving 779 patients with atrial fibrillation found that intravenous magnesium administration led to effective heart rate and rhythm control in 86 per cent of patients compared with 56 per cent in those not receiving magnesium.[54]

Suggested daily dosage: 1.2–10g (but consult an experienced practitioner)

||||||||||||||||||||||||||||||||||||||||||||||||

Chapter 11

THE HEART-HEALTHY LIFESTYLE

If you're looking for the one lifestyle change that will make all the difference to your heart, it's this: do a little exercise every week. This could help to make the difference between your enjoying a healthy, disease-free older age or joining the millions who regularly take an average of 17 prescription drugs every day in the UK.

A pair of researchers from London School of Economics Health discovered exactly how powerful exercise is as a preventative medicine after analyzing 57 trials involving 14,716 people that looked at the benefits of exercise.[1] Not a single trial compared exercise directly with a drug but, through the use of special statistical analyses, they were able to evaluate the benefits of exercise against 248 trials looking at the effects of major pharmaceuticals on chronic conditions such as heart disease, stroke recovery, heart failure and diabetes prevention.

What the researchers discovered wasn't just important – it was revelatory. Plenty of trials have confirmed that exercise is good for us even when we have cancer, arthritis, asthma and/or heart disease, yet none had demonstrated that we could actually throw away the pills.

Those pills – statins, beta blockers, ACE inhibitors, anticoagulants and antiplatelet agents – form the bedrock of the drugs industry. Yet, when assessed against regular exercise, only diuretics, or 'water pills', helped patients with heart failure live longer than they would have done with exercise alone. In fact, for people recovering from stroke, exercise was more beneficial than any drug.

Tantalizingly, this analysis wasn't able to take a more nuanced or detailed look at the type and duration of the exercise – the pooled studies varied widely – but the findings nevertheless highlighted the need to tailor exercise to the given patient.

The researchers were also able to confirm that, whatever the exercise, there's no downside. One Cochrane Collaboration review they cited found no bad reactions to exercise, not even among heart patients who'd been exercising for 10 years or more. And a recent study of people aged 60-plus found that even just moderate exercise once a week may be all we have to do to enjoy a healthy old age.[2]

The armchair generation

Despite all this evidence, far too few of us choose to exercise. In fact, a mere 14 per cent of Britons do any exercise at all, and only 6 per cent get anywhere near enough exercise: half of us do less than 30 minutes of activity a week when we should be doing around 150 minutes a week of moderate exercise, such as taking a brisk walk, cycling, gardening or doing heavy housework. This could be achieved with 21 minutes of exercise every day, or 30 minutes a day for five days a week, giving us two days off.

Your exercise options

What exercise you do, and how vigorously you do it, depends on your age and your mobility. Of course, you can always go to the gym or use a home exercise machine (plan to work out at least 20 minutes a day). But if you're in your late 50s, say, and can still get around reasonably well, here are some alternative simple exercise options:

⇨ **Walking:** Walk at a good pace for 150 minutes a week, or just over 20 minutes a day. If that's too much, then walk at a much gentler pace for eight to 14 hours each week – that's between 68 minutes and two hours every day.

⇨ **Cycling:** Do this for two and a half hours once a week, or halve the time and do it twice a week.

⇨ **Jogging/tennis:** With these more vigorous options, aim for around 75 minutes a week.

⇨ **Ballroom dancing:** You don't have to know how to execute a perfect paso doble to benefit from dancing as long as you do it for at least two hours each week.

⇨ **Mowing the lawn:** This is good for you, but you'll need a very large lawn and grass that grows quickly if mowing is your only exercise. And it has to be the old-fashioned sort of lawnmower that you push around for two hours each week, at least during the growing season or with a lawn that requires mowing all year round.

⇨ **Carrying the groceries:** Lifting anything a little heavy is good muscle-strengthening exercise, and also good for balance and coordination. But remember to lift properly: this means keeping your back straight, flexing your knees and using your legs, not your back. Alternative muscle-strengthening exercises are yoga and serious gardening.

⇨ **A fast swim:** Doing this for 150 minutes each week (or 30 minutes five times) should make the heart work a little harder and leave you a little breathless.

No sweat

Many of us may be put off by the idea of exercise because it conjures up images of sweaty suffering bodies in a gym, but it doesn't have to be quite so punishing, says one new study. Older people who do even a moderate amount of exercise, like walking around the block, are far less likely to suffer a stroke. The key is the length of time you exercise rather than how strenuously you exercise.

According to one study, people who walk for eight to 14 hours a week – at whatever pace – nearly halved their risk of stroke, while those who walked 22 hours a week, or more than three hours every day, had only a third of the stroke risk of people of a similar age who stayed in their armchairs.[3]

In fact, exercise is the number one way to avoid a stroke – and the more you do, the less likely you are to have one. Better yet, it's never too late to start. Men in their late 50s who exercised moderately five days a week – and this can mean just a brisk walk for an hour – reduced their risk of stroke by 46 per cent.[4]

Even if you don't exercise as much as you used to when you were younger, you're still less likely to suffer a stroke than someone who lounged about all those years ago. Early years of vigorous exercise are like money in the bank: it still has a protective effect even if you smoke, or have high blood pressure or a family history of stroke.[5]

Walking towards fitness

Walking at a moderate pace (say 3 miles/hour; 5 km/hour) provides every benefit that running does for staving off degenerative diseases and cardiovascular events.[6] And while most people believe that running or jogging expends more energy than walking, power walking at a pace of at least 5 miles/hour (8 km/hour; or a 12-minute mile) burns more calories than running at a similar speed.[7]

In one study, US researchers looked at data from 72,488 female nurses aged 40 to 65 in 1986 to assess how vigorous exercise has to be to prevent coronary events. What they found, over eight years of follow-up, was that brisk walking was as protective as vigorous exercise, which had long been considered the best choice for preventing coronary heart disease. In fact, walking for three or more hours a week was equivalent to one and a half hours of vigorous exercise, and both were associated with a 30–40 per cent reduction in heart attack risk.[8]

Likewise, in the US Women's Health Initiative Observational Study of 73,743 post-menopausal women, walking was found to be just as good as vigorous exercise for preventing cardiovascular events.[9]

Walking also appears to promote the same oxygen consumption as running or jogging. When sedentary men began a six-month programme of endurance training, those asked to jog six times a week for 30 minutes consumed the same volume of oxygen as walkers walking for the same length of time and frequency. The only difference was that the joggers had higher levels of good HDL cholesterol. A study of previously sedentary women (mean age: 47 years) found that brisk walking decreased heart rate and skin folds (an indicator of fat), and also increased HDL cholesterol.[10]

Even a single walk at a fast pace will improve blood cholesterol levels.[11] Interestingly, exercise intensity doesn't seem to matter when it comes to the amount of fat burned. In a study of men with normal cholesterol levels at UK's Loughborough University, low- and moderate-intensity walking resulted in similar blood fat levels and fat oxidation.[12]

The best news of all is that walking doesn't have to be done all at one time. Whether in one session or accumulated throughout the day, just 30 minutes of brisk walking can reduce blood fats and increase fat-burning.[13] In women, short bouts of brisk walking resulted in similar improvements in fitness and decreases in body fat compared with long bouts, providing that they had the same total duration.[14]

Nevertheless, you should probably go for a brisk walk at least five times a week to get any heart benefits. A bare minimum of 20 minutes three times a week is not enough to lower your risk of cardiovascular disease.[15] Bear in mind that three 10-minute bouts a day are as good as one continuous, 30-minute bout for reducing cardiovascular risk, as well as stress, tension and anxiety.[16]

So, simply deciding to walk more during your day – whether to and from work, to catch the train or get to school, or even just to exercise the dog – can pay big dividends as preventative medicine.

Walking is better than running

Running is undoubtedly hard on the lower limbs. A year-long Australian study found that distance-running injuries were the second most common injury seen at a sports clinic.[17] Runners commonly suffer from overuse injuries of the lower limbs, including stress fractures, and soft tissue injuries such as shin splints, Achilles tendonitis, knee pain and other problems – from simple inflammation to structural degeneration.[18]

The best preventative for such injury is to cut down on your running duration, frequency and/or distance. Also, custom-made biomechanical insoles may reduce shin splints, and a knee brace or support ring can prevent knee pain.[19]

But even walkers have to take care, so here are a few useful tips:

⇨ Walk with your abdominal muscles tightened, and roll back your shoulders, lift your chest, keep your head up and move your arms in a rhythmic swing

⇨ Push off from the toes and land squarely on your heels with each step, then roll from heel to toe

⇨ Make each stride a comfortable length

⇨ Wear good-quality, well-fitting walking shoes or trainers and replace them regularly.

Statin drugs block the benefits of exercise

Statins – and especially simvastatin, marketed as Zocor – block any positive effects that exercise might otherwise have, researchers have found. People who take statins and then start exercising just as the doctor ordered will find their cardiorespiratory (heart and lung) and skeletal-muscle fitness don't get better.

In one study, researchers at Duke University in Durham, North Carolina, monitored 37 people, aged 25 to 59, who were overweight and took no exercise; of these, 18 had also started to take

40mg/day of simvastatin. Even though they all followed the same exercise regime for three months, those taking the statin saw almost no improvement in their risk of the metabolic syndrome – a cluster of factors associated with obesity, cardiovascular disease and type 2 diabetes – while the non-statin group saw a 10 per cent improvement in cardiorespiratory capacity and a 13 per cent increase in skeletal-muscle fitness. In fact, those taking a statin saw a nearly 5 per cent loss in skeletal-muscle capacity in spite of all the exercise.[20]

Other aspects of a healthy lifestyle

All of the following lifestyle practices have been shown to contribute to a healthy heart:

⇨ **Mind–body exercise:** It might be worth incorporating mind–body techniques such as yoga, tai chi and qigong into your daily routine, as they can all help to lower blood pressure.[21] They most likely work by reducing stress and activating the 'relaxation response', that meditative state of deep rest that counteracts the release of stress hormones such as cortisol and adrenaline, especially in men.[22]

⇨ **Sun 'therapy':** Sunlight is our best source of vital vitamin D, which can protect us against all sorts of conditions, including heart disease. As most of us in northern climes are vitamin D-deficient, opt for sensible sun exposure by taking supplements of antioxidants such as selenium, lycopene, beta-carotene and vitamins C and E, all of which offer natural sun protection without the potentially harmful chemicals of sunscreens.

⇨ **Seven hours of sleep:** Two large-scale US surveys found that regularly getting less than six hours or more than nine hours of sleep raised the risk of coronary heart disease, while another study reported a greater risk of stroke with more than eight hours, but not with less than six hours, of sleep. Also, a study of 93,175 post-menopausal women found an increased risk of ischaemic stroke from sleeping less than six hours or more than eight hours every night.[23]

⇨ **Seeking out the new:** Keep your brain active, stay curious and maintain goals – even physical ones. Routine not only deadens the senses, but can actually make us ill. According to Bowling Green State University psychologist Jaak Panksepp, an important basic human instinct is the 'seeking' mode, which drives us to be intensely engaged in the search for answers or solving a puzzle, or just curious about what's new. Every study of longevity shows that those who live to a ripe old age set themselves goals, and remain curious and open to change. A 'pioneering spirit' was apparently the longevity elixir in long-lived American Civil War nurses.[24]

⇨ **Loving your work and working to serve:** Don't settle for anything less than work that makes your heart sing, then do it with gusto. People at peace with their lives and with their life's work live longer than those at war with the world. One of the most fulfilling types of work is living a life of service to others.

⇨ **Erasing old inner emotional tapes:** Thought Field Therapy (TFT) and Emotional Freedom Technique (EFT) are 'needle-free' forms of acupuncture, whereby the therapist or patient 'taps' on points along various meridians of the body while making a series of statements. Both TFT and EFT have been shown to be powerfully effective in overcoming stress from historic events. In patients suffering from post-traumatic stress – a condition considered extremely difficult to treat – TFT reduced such stress by more than half.[25]

⇨ **Cultivating empathy and forgiveness:** One of the greatest antidotes to stress is learning how to forgive, which can help us overcome depression and stress.[26] Gratitude and generosity are two other powerful health-promoting game-changers.

||||||||||||||||||||||||||||||||||||||||||||||

Chapter 12

STAYING CONNECTED

It all started with a chance remark over a couple of beers. A local physician was drinking with the head of medicine at the University of Oklahoma, when he happened to mention that heart disease seemed to be much less common in Roseto, a small town in Pennsylvania close to his surgery, than in neighbouring Bangor.

Roseto's community of 1,600 people was almost entirely made up of transplanted Italians – they even named their small town after the town they'd left behind in Italy – while the 5,000 people in Bangor were an ethnic mix. The two doctors were sure that nationality and ethnic origins had little to do with heart disease, but they were otherwise unable to explain the extraordinary longevity and health rates noted in Roseto.

The name of the physician has since been lost, but the head of medicine was Stewart Wolf, whose name is now synonymous with the 'Roseto effect', as it's come to be known.

Wolf started his research in 1966, when deaths from heart attack and heart disease in Roseto were close to zero among men aged 55 to 64 years – ages at which cardiac mortality was high in the rest of the nation's population. Older Roseto men also fared better than their national counterparts, with a death rate just half of the rest of the country's.

Two other statistics peculiar to Roseto also caught Wolf's eye: the crime rate was close to zero; and applications for public assistance were also non-existent.

But what did all this have to do with heart disease and longevity?

Wolf teamed up with sociologist John Bruhn at Northern Arizona University, who helped him dig a little deeper. Their initial discoveries seemed only to add to the mystery, and flew in the face of government guidelines for heart health.

Virtually all the men in Roseto faced daily hazards as workers in slate quarries that were 200 feet deep, and their diets were appalling. Far from eating the so-called healthy Mediterranean diet, these transplanted Italians were eating sausage and meatballs cooked in lard – in other words, heart-attack food. Not surprisingly, their cholesterol scores were high, with many recording levels up to 200mg/dL (11.11mmol/L); and most were smokers.

The way they lived was also un-American. Three generations of one family lived under one roof, and the elderly members were particularly venerated by the family. Rosetons also seemed to do everything together – evening walks, social clubs, church festivals. In fact, their level of conformity was extraordinary. All displays of wealth – whether through clothing, housing or cars – were strictly taboo, although almost everyone was as poor as everyone else.

The end of the Roseto effect

And this, Wolf and Bruhn realized, wasn't a problem: in fact, it was the reason the Rosetons enjoyed such good health and longevity. This theory was confirmed when the two men looked at the health data, based on analyses of death certificates in both Roseto and Bangor from 1935 to 1985. These revealed that rates of heart attack and longevity began to 'normalize' in Roseto from 1965 onwards, when the town became more prosperous and its citizens moved out into newly built suburbs. By 1985, there were no differences in longevity and heart-attack rates between the two towns.[1]

In a book that Wolf and Bruhn subsequently co-authored, they wrote: 'People are nourished by other people.' In essence, Roseto was a demonstration of the old homily that a problem shared is a problem halved. People supported each other, and there was always someone to turn to, so no one felt isolated, despairing or stressed. A sense of community and sharing was more important for health than lifestyle choices, and could even counteract the effects of smoking, high cholesterol and an unhealthy diet – all factors that would normally contribute to heart disease.[2]

Roseto isn't unique. Many other studies have noted the importance of community in helping people live a long and healthy life, and the phenomenon has been witnessed in groups as diverse as the Amish and social clubs. One study of 230 churchgoers noted they were almost never depressed, even when they had little money or were facing difficult life challenges, so long as they had a strong spiritual belief, but even more importantly, a strong spiritual community.[3]

It appears that collective or communal cultures and societies give their members a tacit or explicit expectation of social support. 'Such support seems to buffer vulnerable individuals from the environmental risks or stressors that serve as triggers to depressive episodes,' said researchers from Northwestern University in Illinois.[4]

Being lonely, getting ill

If community and a sense of belonging are a safeguard against mental and physical disease, then the opposite – social isolation – must be damaging to our health. And countless studies have demonstrated that this is so.

Two studies – one carried out in San Francisco, the other in eastern Finland, and together involving some 20,000 people – revealed that those who felt lonely and lacking in social relationships and support were up to three times more likely to die of heart disease and other causes than those who felt connected to others. And just as the Roseto researchers found, having a social connection, or not, was a more powerful agent of wellness and disease than the usual risk factors of high cholesterol, hypertension, smoking and a family history of heart disease.[5]

So, living alone or feeling isolated is like smoking 15 cigarettes a day or being an alcoholic, and twice as harmful as obesity. Researchers at Brigham Young University in Utah arrived at these conclusions after analyzing 148 studies of the relationship between frequency of human interaction and overall health over a seven-year period. In contrast, having social connections and ties with friends, family, neighbours and the wider community had a protective effect and improved the chances of survival by 50 per cent.[6]

In fact, the researchers believed that the protective effect might be even greater, but decided to take a more conservative view. Likewise, the harmful effects of isolation may also be much worse.

'Physicians, health professionals, educators and the media take risk factors such as smoking, diet and exercise seriously. The data presented here make a compelling case for social-relationship factors to be added to that list,' said lead researcher Timothy Smith.

Other studies have revealed that:

⇨ People with three or fewer people in their social support network are more than twice as likely to die of heart disease – or any other disease – than people with larger social networks. As the Roseto studies showed, isolation has a greater impact on health than the usual hazards like smoking, say researchers from Duke University Medical Center in North Carolina, after examining the social profiles of 430 patients with coronary artery disease.[7]

⇨ Loneliness builds up over time, say researchers at the University of Chicago. They found a direct correlation, over four years, between blood pressure and periods of loneliness and, in particular, a sense of being alone.[8]

⇨ Being socially isolated – and feeling alone – doubles the risk of death from a cardiovascular disease or any other cause, say Canadian researchers. The risk disappeared in those who never felt alone regardless of whether they actually lived on their own or not.[9]

⇨ Social isolation has a greater impact on men than on women, according to a study that measured blood levels of leptin, a marker of cardiovascular disease. In 1,229 men and women, social isolation significantly raised leptin in men, but not in women, said researchers from Munich, Germany.[10] But even in women, being in a long-term relationship made dying of ischaemic heart disease 28 per cent less likely than in single women, according to an Oxford University study.[11]

It's now indisputable that social isolation is a major cause of chronic disease, especially heart problems. California heart expert Dr Dean Ornish has uncovered an extraordinary statistic: all the usual risk factors for heart disease – smoking, obesity, sedentary lifestyle and a high-fat diet – only account for half of all heart disease. In Ornish's research, no risk factor appears more dangerous than simple isolation – from other people, from our own feelings and from a 'higher power'.

Studies of other populations, such as Japanese Americans, have also demonstrated that social networks and social support protect them against coronary heart disease and heart attack – regardless of smoking or high blood pressure.[12] What these men ate – be it tofu and sushi or a Big Mac – had no bearing on their propensity for heart disease so long as they maintained strong social ties.

The mind–body connection

What's less clear is *how* this happens: in other words, the actual biological mechanism(s) that loneliness triggers to cause disease.

For cognitive disorders such as Alzheimer's disease, the association may be easier to grasp. It's been noted that older people who feel isolated and lonely are twice as likely to develop the disease as those who maintain a social network. As the researchers concluded, 'It may be that loneliness may affect systems in the brain dealing with cognition and memory, making lonely people more vulnerable to the effects of age-related decline in neural pathways.'[13]

Researchers at the Harvard School of Public Health believe that isolation can lead to inflammatory problems, possibly due to changes in the immune system. Virtually all the lonely people they assessed (who were from the Framingham Heart Study) had raised levels of C-reactive protein (CRP) and fibrinogen, and especially interleukin (IL-6), all of which were markers of inflammation.[14] It may be that lonely people are simply generating more stress hormones, say researchers at the University of Chicago, and this encourages tumour growth, especially in cases of breast cancer.

According to Dr Caryn Lerman, deputy editor of the journal *Cancer Prevention Research*, which published the Chicago study, 'This study shows that social isolation alters expression of genes important in mammary-gland tumour growth.'[15]

Professor Thea Tisty, at the University of California at San Francisco, believes that the Chicago study adds to the growing evidence of a causal connection between isolation and chemicals in the blood such as stress hormones, which could be turning genes on and off within cells, leading to all manner of serious illness.[16]

How lonely is lonely?

Feeling lonely is an entirely subjective experience. Some people may have a wide circle of friends and still feel lonely, while others may have just one or two friends and feel part of a community.

Marriage, or a monogamous partnership of some sort, is the single most important relationship most of us have, and the sense of closeness we feel with our partner can determine our sense of isolation or connection.

We may then feel so isolated when our partner dies that it kills us, a phenomenon known as the 'widowhood effect'. Researchers at St Andrew's University in Scotland tracked nearly 60,000 men and the same number of women who were married in 1991. Over the following 15 years, nearly a tenth of the men and almost twice that number of women lost their partners, and of these people, 40 per cent of widowers and 36 per cent of widows died within three years of their loss.

Although the deaths were put down to various causes, the researchers found that the widowhood effect – the sudden realization of being alone – was the common factor shared by those who'd died.[17] While the surviving partner may have had a wide and supportive network, the loss of 'the significant other' was paramount.

The Scottish researchers concluded that some people give up on life within six months of losing a partner, and that the broken heart syndrome can persist many months or even years after bereavement.

Most interesting of all was that the actual cause of death didn't seem to matter. The departed partners had died of illnesses like cancer or heart attack, self-inflicted causes such as alcohol abuse, smoking or suicide, accidents such as a car crash, and even murder. It was as though, once a partner was gone, the remaining spouse felt left behind and simply decided to give up.

In fact, this syndrome is not confined to humans: a similar situation is found among animals. Researchers conducting heart studies on rabbits were flabbergasted to find that, among the animals given high-cholesterol-producing diets, those who were played with and petted by the researchers developed less cardiovascular disease than those stuck in cages out of reach and left alone.

Another study has suggested that the most important factor in counteracting loneliness isn't a social network *per se*, but how much support it offers. This means that a supportive network of just one or two people, while not as heart-protective as a larger group, can be enough to make someone feel connected and part of a community, say researchers at the University of Michigan in Ann Arbor.[18]

Being lonely is often associated with being old, especially after a partner dies and the survivor is incapacitated in some way. Yet the truth is that feelings of isolation cut across all population groups and ages. The Brigham Young University researchers, who concluded that social isolation was equivalent to smoking 15 cigarettes a day, also found that it affected all age groups. 'This effect is not isolated to older adults. Relationships provide a level of protection across all ages,' said lead researcher Timothy Smith.

Even kids aren't immune. Children as young as five who feel isolated and alone are far more likely to have heart disease as an adult. According to research by the University of Wisconsin, which followed the progress of 1,037 children into adulthood, those who'd been socially isolated were far more likely to have cardiovascular disease or be candidates for it, with raised blood pressure, higher cholesterol and/or obesity, by the age of 26.[19]

An actual broken heart

Several years ago, Hollywood was shocked when actress Brittany Murphy, just 32, died of pneumonia, which she contracted after taking over-the-counter drugs. Within five months, her doting husband, British screenwriter Simon Monjack, aged 40, was also dead. He'd died from cardiac arrest – his heart had literally broken.

Scientists have tried to explain the widowhood effect as due to the similar lifestyles between couples who are then, as a consequence, exposed to the same risk factors. But Japanese cardiologists arrived at a better explanation after discovering the phenomenon of 'stress cardiomyopathy'. This happens when a deep emotional stress – resulting from a sudden break-up, rejection, death of a partner, or even work-related or financial worries – causes dysfunction in the ventricular chamber and heart failure in people with no signs of cardiovascular disease.[20] In these cases, now dubbed 'broken-heart syndrome', heart muscle cells (myocytes) suffer degenerative changes leading to cell death.

Researchers at Johns Hopkins University in Baltimore, Maryland, found that women with this syndrome had none of the usual predisposing factors of heart disease. What they'd suffered was purely psychological, from the stress of break-up or the death of a loved one. Yet the bereavement or sadness had released such toxic levels of stress hormones, particularly adrenaline, that they'd 'stunned' the heart, literally causing it to 'break'.[21]

Believe in something

Many things can bring about feelings of isolation and loneliness. It may be the death of a partner or loved one, or chronic depression, or just a generally pessimistic view of the world and mankind. Ultimately, this adds up to a profound feeling of disconnectedness and hopelessness – a sense of being utterly alone.

Not surprisingly, having a religious or philosophical belief that we're all connected can have beneficial effects on our health and wellbeing, regardless of a strong social network. Indeed, those with strong religious beliefs are better able to cope following a stroke, as one study found. Stroke patients who had religious or spiritual beliefs had less anxiety and depression than those who were agnostic or atheist.[22]

Religious beliefs also helped to prevent Croatian war veterans from committing suicide. Those who had strong religious convictions also had less chronic post-traumatic stress than those with no faith.[23]

What's more, it may be enough just to have these beliefs privately without belonging to a wider community of fellow believers, such as a church congregation. As one study found, people who held religious or spiritual beliefs without belonging to any organized religion enjoyed better mental equilibrium than those without a spiritual belief system.[24] This also translates into a heart-healthy effect; Norwegian research has shown that people who go to church most Sundays have much lower blood pressure than those who rarely, or never, attend.[25]

Non-religious spiritual beliefs that make people feel connected to something greater also include forgiveness and empathy. Those who learned how to forgive and empathize with others had dramatically lower levels of depression and stress after a year.[26]

Is your glass half-full?

Does loneliness make us pessimistic and 'down', or is a pessimistic outlook the cause of our loneliness?

We now know that cheerful and optimistic people are far less likely to have heart attacks. All positive moods – like happiness, and feeling relaxed, energetic and generally good about your life – play a big part in determining whether you'll have heart disease.

Researchers at Johns Hopkins University School of Medicine tracked the health of 1,483 people whose siblings had been afflicted with a heart problem before the age of 60. According to genetics, the sibling of a heart patient should be twice as likely to develop the condition as someone with a healthy brother or sister. But in the study this risk was reduced in siblings who had a happy outlook on life, falling by one-third, and in some cases to 50 per cent.[27]

Learning to be optimistic is something we can all work on, says American psychologist Martin Seligman, the inventor of 'positive psychology', which examines the emotional states that make for a longer and happier life. Negative thoughts are often knee-jerk unconscious responses to problems or setbacks. You can work on them by:

⇨ Keeping a journal of any negative thoughts you have

⇨ Looking for patterns (what situations make you think the worst?)

⇨ Giving yourself credit when something good happens to you, and not beating yourself up when bad things happen.[28]

Getting connected

Many techniques and lifestyle choices can help to overcome loneliness and its worst effects. Here are a few ways to get connected:

⇨ **Meditation:** This practice can help you feel connected to a higher power and reduce levels of stress. There are many forms of meditation, from focused intoning of a sound (mantra) or concentrating on a spiritual pattern (mandala) to mindfulness meditation (non-judgmental awareness of present-moment experiences). Several techniques have been tested for treating heart conditions, all with highly positive results. Transcendental Meditation (TM) – which involves repeating a mantra – can reduce the early-stage symptoms of raised blood pressure, reduce the chances of a fatal heart problem by nearly a third and lower the risk of death from cancer by nearly half.[29]

When TM was tested in 201 men and women with an average age of 59 with long-standing heart disease, half were instructed in TM, which they performed for 20 minutes twice a day, while the rest were given advice on modifying their diet and exercising regularly. The TM group saw such a dramatic improvement in their condition that the researchers reckoned they reduced their risk of dying from a heart attack or stroke by 48 per cent, compared to the controls.[30]

'If TM were a drug conferring so many benefits, it would be a billion-dollar blockbuster,' said research team leader Norman Rosenthal, then from the US National Institute of Mental Health.

⇨ **Touch therapy:** This healing technique involves contact, an obvious and palpable way to connect, and it seems to have the same beneficial effects as having a positive outlook, and a general sense of caring and empathy. When having such feelings and touching, the body releases oxytocin – a powerful cardiovascular hormone also known as the 'love' or 'trust' hormone – which reduces stress and lowers blood pressure.[31]

⇨ **Massage therapy:** One of the most powerful touch therapies is massage, which can reduce anxiety and depression while increasing vitality and general health.[32]

Chapter 13

AT-A-GLANCE TIPS FOR A HEALTHY HEART

Here's a quick-reference checklist drawn from the facts and observations outlined in this book. If you've had any history of heart problems, follow this programme only under the supervision of a qualified, experienced professional. Also, consult a professional with good knowledge of nutrition about the doses of supplements to take, since these vary, depending on your individual needs.

For Healthy People and All Heart Patients

⇨ Keep a healthy body weight. Ignore the recommendations for calculating your ideal weight using the BMI (body mass index), a clumsy method of calculating weight status that has no relation to heart health.

⇨ Don't smoke.

⇨ Follow the Mediterranean-style diet, which is rich in fruits and vegetables and olive oil, with meat as a condiment, rather than the centrepiece of meals.

⇨ Avoid high-GI foods like white bread, potatoes, freshly made pastas and sugary snacks, biscuits and cakes.

⇨ Eat fish liberally, but choose carefully to avoid consuming harmful contaminants like mercury and dioxins. Avoid fish from the North Sea, deep-water fish and farmed fish.

⇨ Eat whole, unprocessed, organic foods grown locally and in season and cooked by traditional methods.

⇨ Eat organic eggs liberally.

⇨ Eat more legumes such as well-cooked (several hours or more) lentils and kidney beans.

⇨ Avoid all hydrogenated margarine and other hydrogenated oils, but don't limit saturated fats.

⇨ Engage in regular exercise, ideally 20 minutes a day.

⇨ Take foods and supplements high in omega-3 fatty acids, such as fish or flaxseed oils.

   Daily dosage for supplements: 1,000–1,500mg omega-3 fatty acids as fish or flaxseed oil

⇨ Drink red wine in moderation – one or two glasses a day seems to be protective (but avoid, of course, if you're pregnant).

⇨ Drink green tea regularly.

⇨ Eat a square or two of dark chocolate daily.

⇨ Snack regularly on heart-healthy nuts such as walnuts, pecans and almonds.

⇨ Fast occasionally.

⇨ Ditch homogenized or low-fat dairy produce.

⇨ Take a good-quality multivitamin/mineral supplement produced by a reputable manufacturer.

⇨ Make sure you're getting enough of the B vitamins, especially B6 (100mg/day), B1 (50mg/day) and B3 (50mg/day).

⇨ Maintain good intake of the antioxidant vitamins – vitamins A (up to 25,000IU as beta-carotene or 10,000IU as retinol), C (1–3g/day or more) and E (1–3g/day or up to 600IU as tocotrienols – as well as zinc (10–50mg/day) and selenium (200mcg/day).

⇨ Get a daily dose of chromium (100mcg) and magnesium (200–600mg), both important for heart health.

⇨ Take other heart-healthy supplements: CoQ 10 (60–100mg/day or more with supervision); l-carnitine (250–750mg/day)

⇨ Don't forget vitamin D, which you can get naturally by exposing your skin to the sun for about 15 minutes early in the day without sunscreen, or supplement with 600–1,000IU/day.

⇨ Take a high-quality probiotic supplement (most good ones are sold refrigerated).

⇨ Get seven hours' sleep a night – the optimal amount for the heart.

⇨ Engage in a regular relaxation exercise that has been shown to lower blood pressure and calm the heart – TM, biofeedback, meditation and the like.

⇨ Enjoy your life. Change your job or any other part of your life if you don't like it.

⇨ Work on ending isolation from your own feelings, from other people or from a higher power. Making friends, expressing your feelings, taking care of a pet, praying or developing your own spirituality may save your life.

⇨ Love and be loved.

For Specific Conditions

For furred-up arteries

⇨ Try chelation therapy, which chemically 'grabs' hardened plaque, administered by a qualified, experienced professional.

⇨ Get needled. Acupuncture has been proven to increase the work capacity of hearts.

⇨ Take blue-green algae, shown to help clean up blocked arteries.

⇨ Go to a herbalist, who may prescribe bromelain, ginger, *Ginkgo biloba* or *Terminalia arjuna* – all have been shown to work.

⇨ Check out Chinese herbs, particularly *Andrographis paniculata* Nees, known in Indian Ayurvedic medicine as *Bhui-neem*.

⇨ Opt for gugulipid, the Ayurvedic remedy, which helps prevent atherosclerosis.

For angina

⇨ Take the pineapple enzyme bromelain – 125 to 450mg three times a day.

⇨ Consult a qualified herbalist to prescribe herbs such as *Khella* or extract of barberry root.

⇨ Increase your intake of thiamine (take 50mg/day). Low levels of this B vitamin also increase your heart attack risk.

⇨ Take Coenzyme Q10, or CoQ10 (150mg/day), as this can reduce the frequency of angina attacks.

⇨ Try homeopathy. Tinctures of *Crataegus oxyacantha* (hawthorn) may protect the heart after an angina attack.

For hypertension

⇨ Keep your weight down. Losing weight, if you're overweight, will lower blood pressure naturally.

⇨ Engage in regular exercise, at least 20 minutes per day.

⇨ Avoid processed carbs and try to eat mainly low-GI foods.

⇨ Avoid the Pill and NSAIDs such as ibuprofen, which raise blood pressure.

⇨ Take a heavy metals blood test to check your levels of lead and cadmium, which can cause hypertension. (These are given by Genova Diagnostics: see www.gdx.net, which has both UK and US webpages.)

⇨ Cook with traditional fats such as coconut oil or butter or cold-pressed (traditionally pressed without heating) olive oil.

⇨ Limit alcohol to one drink per day.

⇨ Eat potassium-rich foods such as bananas or take a potassium supplement, which will help to lower blood pressure dramatically.

⇨ Take magnesium (200–600mg/day), which may also help to lower blood pressure.

⇨ Get enough calcium in your food. Low levels of calcium may bring on hypertension. Make sure your levels of vitamin D3 are adequate to ensure better uptake of calcium.

⇨ Take CoQ10 supplements to bring down blood pressure. Try 150mg/day.

⇨ Consider taking relevant herbal preparations. Try *Achillea Wilhelmsii* extract (15–20 drops twice daily) or tomato extract (15mg of lycopene). Other good herbs include barberry root bark, extract from *Ammi visnaga* or the Ayurvedic combo medicine *Abana*.

⇨ Pop homeopathic Cytisus Laburnum at 6 DH potency twice daily.

⇨ Make time for relaxation or mind–body techniques, particularly yoga, TM or the Chinese therapy qigong.

⇨ Explore hypnosis with a qualified, experienced practitioner.

⇨ Consider acupuncture.

To prevent stroke

⇨ Eat at least five portions of fruit and vegetables daily.

⇨ Consume 1–2 glasses of red wine (or red grape juice, which gives the same benefit) daily.

⇨ Eat plenty of walnuts, soya and rapeseed or canola oil – all good sources of omega-3 fatty acids.

⇨ Start exercising today and get your children exercising early in life.

⇨ Keep antioxidant vitamins A, C and E levels high, with the same dosages recommended for general heart patients, but don't take more than 400mg/day of vitamin E without the supervision of an experienced, qualified practitioner.

⇨ Take B vitamins, which reduce levels of homocysteine.

Suggested daily dosage: 1mg folate as L-methylfolate or vitamin B9, 10mg B6, 400mcg B12

⇨ Take supplements of garlic (800mg/day of garlic powder) and *Gingko biloba* (120–600mg/day), both powerful natural blood thinners.

⇨ Eat raw ginger: about 5g daily. This can lower blood-clotting agents in the blood.

⇨ Try qigong, an ancient Chinese form of exercise that's particularly effective for slashing stroke risk.

If you've already had a heart attack

⇨ Take l-carnitine (250–750mg/day), which will help protect you from future attacks.

⇨ Take Coenzyme Q10 (60–100mg/day), which can prevent heartbeat irregularities and the tissue damage usually seen after a heart attack.

⇨ Eat a few squares of dark chocolate every day.

⇨ Ask your doctor about intravenous infusions of magnesium, given soon after a heart attack. These have been shown to work as well as thrombolysis or antiplatelet therapy but without the side-effects.

⇨ Increase your levels of antioxidants, which can reduce the possibility of future heart attacks (although the results of some studies are mixed). Follow dosages given under general advice for heart patients, above.

⇨ Consider taking higher levels of vitamin B6 (take more than 100mg per day only with medical supervision) to protect your heart from further damage.

⇨ Take thiamine supplements indefinitely after a heart attack (same dosages as for general heart patients) to help your heart's ventricular function improve.

After heart surgery

⇨ Consider acupuncture as a way to help alleviate pain and regulate your heart afterwards.

⇨ Take the Chinese herb *Andrographis paniculata* Nees after coronary angioplasty: it helps to prevent restenosis (re-narrowing of arteries).

For heart flutters

⇨ Avoid potential dietary triggers, such as caffeine, wheat, dairy, sweeteners and artificial additives.

⇨ Be wary of painkillers, which can raise your risk of atrial fibrillation.

⇨ Try intravenous magnesium under the supervision of an experienced practitioner.

⇨ Consider acupuncture, which can work wonders for heart rhythm problems, especially when H5, H7 and H8 acupoints are needed.

⇨ Try Scotch broom, an effective non-toxic herbal medicine.

Suggested dosage: 1tbsp (10ml) three or four times a day

⇨ Try homeopathy, which has several remedies suitable for atrial fibrillation, including homeopathic Scotch broom (2DH), Hoitzia Coccinea (3DH) and Hydrophis Cyanocinctus (4CH).

Suggested daily dosage: 2DH

|||||||||||||||||||||||||||||||||||||||||||

REFERENCES

Part I: The Myth of Prevention

Chapter 1: The Myth about Fats and Cholesterol

1. Nutr Metab Cardiovasc Dis, 2012; 22: 1039–45
2. J Gerontol A Biol Sci Med Sci, 2007; 62: 1164–71
3. Am J Physiol, 1954; 178: 30–2
4. Keys A. *Seven Countries: A Multivariate Analysis of Death and Coronary Heart Disease*. Cambridge, MA/London: Harvard University Press, 1980
5. Science, 2001; 291: 2536–45
6. Quart J Med, 2003; 96: 927–34
7. JAMA, 1987; 257: 2176–80
8. JAMA, 1994; 272: 1335–40
9. www.health.harvard.edu/fhg/updates/ update1104b.shtml
10. Arch Intern Med, 2006; 145: 520–30
11. www.saintthomasheart.com/cholesterol
12. Am Heart J, 2009; 157: 111–7.e2
13. Am J Clin Nutr, 2010; 91: 502–9
14. Nutrition, 2012; 28: 118–23
15. Ann Intern Med, 2014; 160: 398–406
16. BMJ, 2000; 321: 199–204
17. Circulation, 1992; 86: 1046–60
18. Ann Hematol, 2008; 87: 223–8
19. Lancet, 1997; 350: 1119–23
20. J Gerontol A Biol Sci Med Sci, 2010; 65: 559–64
21. www.heartmdinstitute.com/126–hmd–root/hmd–articles/399–worried–about–cholesterol

22. Lancet, 1997; 350: 1119–23

23. BMJ, 1994; 309: 11–5

24. N Engl J Med, 1977; 297: 644–50

Chapter 2: The Myth of Dangerous Blood Pressure Levels

1. JAMA, 2014; 311: 507–20

2. Heart, 2014; 100: 456–64

3. Drugs Aging, 2003; 20: 277–86

4. J Gen Intern Med, 2011; 26: 685–90

5. Lancet, 2000; 355: 865–72

6. J Hypertens, 2006: 24: 459–62

7. J Am Coll Cardiol, 2001; 37: 163–8

8. Acad Emerg Med, 2004; 11: 237–43

9. Engl J Med, 1985; 312: 1548–51

10. J Manag Care Pharm, 2007; 13 [suppl S–b]: S34–9

11. Lancet, 2007; 370: 1219–29

12. Arch Intern Med, 2007; 167: 388–93; JAMA, 1995; 274: 1343

Chapter 3: Aspirin to Prevent Stroke: Spin, Not Science

1. Lancet, 1992; 339: 342–4

2. BMC Med, 2009; 7: 53

3. BMJ, 1995; 311: 139–40

4. Lancet Neurol, 2007; 6: 487–93

5. Health Technol Assess, 2013; 17: 1–253

6. Gastroenterology Insights, 2013; 5: e3

7. Hospital Medicine, 1995; 31: 29

Chapter 4: The Unhealthy Plate

1. Lancet, 1957; 273: 959–66

2. Am J Clin Nutr, 2005; 81: 1147–54; Acta Oncol, 2012; 51: 454–64

3. Am J Public Health, 1997; 87: 992–7

4. J Clin Epidemiol, 1998; 51: 443–60

5. Enig MG, Fallon S. *The Skinny on Fats*. The Weston A. Price Foundation, 2000; www.westonaprice.org/know–your–fats/skinny–on–fats

6. J Natl Cancer Inst, 1986; 77: 43–51

7. Lancet, 1993; 341: 75–9; Br J Psychiatry, 2000; 176: 399–400

8. Curr Med Res Opin, 2005; 21: 95–100

9. J Am Phys Surg, 2004; 9: 109–13

10. Am J Clin Nutr, 2000; 71: 682–92
11. 'Characteristics of Traditional Diets'; www.westonaprice.org/basics/characteristics–of–traditional–diets
12. J Clin Endocrinol Metab, 2003; 88: 1617–23
13. Am J Clin Nutr, 1983; 37: 740–8
14. Curr Atheroscler Rep, 2010; 12: 384–90; Am J Clin Nutr, 2010; 91: 1541–2
15. http://ornishspectrum.com/proven–program/nutrition/
16. Food Chem, 2011; 129: 155–61
17. J Agric Food Chem, 2009; 57: 471–7
18. JAMA, 1999; 281: 1387–94
19. Biol Res, 2003; 36: 291–302
20. Am J Clin Nutr, 1994; 60: 973–4
21. Rogers S. *Wellness Against All Odds*. Prestige Pubs, 1994
22. Curr Opin Endocrinol Diabetes Obes, 2009; 16: 163–71
23. Eur J Clin Nutr, 1998; 52: 334–43; Am J Clin Nutr, 1999; 69: 403–10
24. Atherosclerosis, 1986; 61: 219–23
25. Lakartidningen, 1998; 95: 5146–8
26. J Nutr Med, 1991; 2: 227–47
27. N Engl J Med, 1991; 325: 1704–8
28. J Nutr Med, 1991; 2: 227–47

Chapter 5: The True Causes of Heart Disease

1. JAMA Intern Med, 2014; 174: 516–24
2. J Gen Intern Med, 2012; 27: 1120–6
3. Presented at the American Stroke Association International Stroke Conference, February 9–11, 2011, Los Angeles, CA
4. Annu Rev Med, 1998; 49: 235–61
5. Diabetes Technol Ther, 2006; 8: 677–87
6. BMJ Open Heart, 2014; 1: e000032
7. Ann Intern Med, 2014; 160: 398–406
8. JAMA, 1996; 275: 759
9. Lancet, 1994; 343: 1268–71
10. J Lipid Res, 1992; 33: 399–410
11. Lancet, 1993; 341: 581–5
12. Br J Prev Soc Med, 1975; 29: 82–90
13. www.chekinstitute.com/freegifts847386/DoesFatMakeYouFat.pdf
14. www.nhlbi.nih.gov/files/docs/resources/heart/atp3full.pdf
15. Lancet, 1995; 345: 273–8
16. EMBO Mol Med, 2014; 6: 744–59

17. Circ Heart Fail, 2014; 7: 552–7

18. Lancet, 2004; 364: 937–52

19. Arterioscler Thromb, 1994; 14: 54–9

20. J Periodontol, 2008; 79 [8 Suppl]: 1544–51

21. N Engl J Med, 2005; 352: 20–8

22. BMJ, 2000; 321: 199–204

23. Am J Pathol, 1969; 56: 111–28

24. JAMA, 1995; 274: 1049–57

25. N Engl J Med, 1995; 332: 286–91

26. JAMA, 1992; 268: 877–81

27. N Engl J Med, 1997; 337: 230–6

28. Eur J Cardiovasc Prev Rehabil, 2009; 16: 150–5

29. J Periodontol, 2008; 79: 1652–8

30. www.dentalhealth.org/news/details/457

31. Stroke, 2004; 35: 496–501

32. Stroke, 2003; 34: 47–52

33. Atherosclerosis, 2010; 213: 263–7

34. Ann Periodontol, 2003; 8: 38–53

35. J Am Dent Assoc, 2002; 133 Suppl: 14S–22S

36. Ann Periodontol, 2001; 6: 125–37

37. Arthritis Res Ther, 2010; 12: 218

38. Alzheimers Dement, 2008; 4: 242–50

39. Curr Opin Nephrol Hypertens, 2010; 19: 519–26

40. FASEB J, 2009; 23: 1196–204

41. Altern Med Rev, 1996; 1: 11–7

42. Altern Med Rev, 1996; 1: 11–7

43. Clin Diagn Lab Immunol, 2003; 10: 897–902

44. Int J Vitam Nutr Res, 1982; 52: 333–41

45. J Am Diet Assoc, 2010; 110: 1669–75

46. JAMA, 2003; 290: 2945–51

47. JAMA, 1994; 272: 781–6

48. Am J Hyptertens, 2010; 23: 1031–7

Part II: Standard Medical Treatment

Chapter 6: Statin Wonderland

1. Open J Endocrine Metabol Dis, 2013; 3: 179–85

2. Kendrick M. *The Great Cholesterol Con: The Truth About What Really Causes Heart Disease and How to Avoid It*. London: John Blake Publishing, 2007

3. Open J Endocrine Metabol Dis, 2013; 3; 179–85
4. Lancet, 2001; 358: 351–5
5. JAMA, 1987; 257: 2176–80
6. N Engl J Med, 2007; 357: 2109–22
7. Lancet, 2001; 358: 351–5
8. JAMA, 1994; 272: 1335–40
9. BMJ, 1992; 304: 431–3
10. BMJ, 1995; 310: 1632–6
11. Lancet, 1992; 339: 727–9
12. Lancet, 1993; 341: 75–9
13. Psychol Med, 1990; 20: 785–91
14. Werbach M. *Nutritional Influences on Mental Illness.* Tarzana, CA: Third Line Press, 1991: 145–9
15. Eur J Prev Cardiol, 2014; 21: 464–74
16. Lancet, 1994; 344: 1383–9
17. N Engl J Med, 1995; 333: 1301–7
18. BMJ, 2008; 336: 180–1
19. Mov Disord, 2007; 22: 377–81
20. N Engl J Med, 2008; 359: 789–99
21. Kendrick M. *The Great Cholesterol Con.* London: John Blake Publishing, 2007

Chapter 7: Other Heart Drugs

1. Eur Heart J, 2004; 25: 2019–25
2. Circulation, 1986; 74:1124–36
3. Circulation, 1991; 83:1084–6
4. J Am Coll Cardiol, 1994; 24: 1133–42
5. Vasc Health Risk Manag, 2007; 3: 629–37; J Am Coll Cardiol, 1997; 30: 947–54
6. JAMA, 2012; 308: 1340–9
7. J Am Coll Cardiol, 2000; 36: 147–50
8. Lancet, 1996; 347: 1056
9. JAMA, 1996; 275: 423–4
10. N Engl J Med, 1991; 324: 781–8
11. Lancet, 1996; 348: 7–12
12. Sci Transl Med, 2011; 3: 107ra111
13. N Engl J Med, 1997; 336: 525–33
14. Circ Cardiovasc Qual Outcomes, 2013; 6: 525–33
15. N Engl J Med, 1996; 335: 1253–60
16. Lancet, 1994; 343: 311–22
17. N Engl J Med, 2005; 352: 1637–45, 1646–54

18. Circulation, 1997; 95: 2075–81

19. N Engl J Med, 1989; 320: 709–18

20. Hope R-E. *Worse Pills, Best Pills II*. Washington, DC: Public Citizen's Health Research Group, 1993: 10

21. Lancet, 1994; 344: 1019–20

22. J Am Coll Cardiol, 1999; 34: 1360–2

23. J Hum Hypertens, 2010; 24: 336–44

24. Circulation, 2008; 117: 2706–15

25. J Hypertens, 2007; 25: 1751–62

26. JAMA, 1995; 274: 620–5

27. BMJ, 2010; 340: c103

28. Lancet, 2005; 366: 1545–53

29. BMJ, 2004; 329: 1248–9

30. JAMA, 2003; 289: 2534–44

31. Heart, 2014; 100: 456–64

32. http://loisrogers.com/health/800000-killed-by-beta-blockers/

33. Hypertension, 1994; 24: 480–5

34. J Hum Hypertens, 1994; 8: 233–7; Am J Kidney Dis, 1994; 23: 471–5

35. Am J Hypertens,1991; 4: 468–71

36. Ceska Gynekol, 1994; 59: 62–3

37. Am J Hypertens, 1993; 6: 287–94

38. Br J Clin Pharmacol, 1993; 35: 455–9

39. Am J Cardiol, 1992; 70: 1306–9

40. DICP, 1991; 25: 1068–70

41. JAMA, 1995; 274: 1839–45

42. BMJ, 1996; 312: 83–8

43. Fundam Clin Pharmacol, 2004;18: 139–51; Am J Cardiol, 2002; 90: 1050–5

44. Eur Heart J, 1998; 19: 1758–65

45. Intensive Care Med, 1995; 21: 82–3

46. Rev Clin Esp, 1993; 192: 228–30

47. BMJ, 1992; 305: 693

48. Am J Clin Oncol, 1992; 15: 168–73

49. Acta Neurol Belg, 1992; 92: 45–7

50. Lancet, 1991; 338: 1158

51. J Neurol Neurosurg Psychiatry; 1989; 52: 541–3

52. Med J Aust, 1987; 146: 412–4

53. Am J Emerg Med, 1987; 5: 163–4

54. South Med J, 1995; 88: 352–4; Eur Neurol, 1994; 34: 16–22

55. Neurology, 1994; 44: 2405–6

56. Circulation, 1995; 92: 2811–8
57. Circulation; 1991; 83: 448–59
58. Arch Neurol, 1985; 42: 1033
59. Stroke, 1994; 25: 1065–7
60. Nervenarzt, 1994; 65: 125–7
61. Stroke, 1996; 27: 1033–9
62. Eur Heart J, 2014; 35: 1881–7
63. Circ Cardiovasc Qual Outcomes, 2011; 4: 14–21
64. Stroke, 2000; 31: 1555–60
65. N Engl J Med, 1995; 333: 1581–8
66. Lancet, 1995; 346: 1509–14
67. JAMA, 1995; 274: 1017–25
68. Circulation, 1995; 92: 2811–8
69. BMJ, 1994; 308: 81–106; 159–68; 235–46
70. Br Med J [Clin Res Ed], 1988; 296: 320–31
71. J Indian Acad Clin Med, 2003; 4: 315–22
72. Am J Med, 2011; 124: 426–33
73. BMJ, 1994; 308: 71–73
74. QuarterWatch, 2012; www.ismp.org/quarterwatch/pdfs/2011Q4.pdf
75. Circulation, 2012; 126: 1955–63
76. PLoS Med, 2011 Sep; 8 (9): e1001098.d
77. Circulation, 2011; 123: 2226–35
78. Am J Med, 2011; 124: 614–20
79. N Engl J Med, 2004; 351: 2611–8
80. http://shared.web.emory.edu/whsc/news/releases/2011/04/antidepressants–linked–to–thicker–arteries.html
81. BMJ, 2014; 349: g4930
82. N Engl J Med, 2012; 366: 1881–90

Chapter 8: Operations for Heart Disease

1. N Engl J Med, 2012; 366: 1467–76
2. JAMA, 2011; 306: 2128–36
3. J Am Coll Cardiol, 2011; 58: 1426–32
4. Arch Intern Med, 2012; 172: 112–7
5. Vasc Health Risk Manag, 2006; 2: 477–84
6. J Am Coll Cardiol, 1997; 30: 1451–60
7. JAMA, 1996; 276: 300–6
8. Ann Intern Med, 2001; 135: 616–32
9. Stroke, 1999; 30: 514–22

10. JAMA, 2002; 287: 1405–12
11. Stroke, 2000; 31: 707–13
12. Anesth Analg, 2004; 98: 1610–7
13. Eur J Cardiothorac Surg, 2010; 37: 112–8
14. N Engl J Med, 2004; 350: 21–8
15. N Engl J Med, 2012; 366: 1467–76
16. Circulation, 2013; 127: 1656–63
17. Medicina [Kaunas], 2007; 43: 183–9
18. N Engl J Med, 2007; 356: 1009–19
19. Eur Heart J, 1997; 18, 1536–47
20. J Invasive Cardiol, 2013; 25: E114–9
21. J Am Coll Cardiol, 2013; 62: B6–B6
22. EuroIntervention, 2011; 7: 872–7
23. JAMA, 2011; 306: 53–61
24. N Engl J Med, 2007; 356: 1503–16
25. N Engl J Med, 1993; 329: 221–7
26. Eur Heart J, 2000; 21: 1759–66
27. Cochrane Database Syst Rev, 2010; 3: CD004815
28. N Engl J Med, 1998; 338: 1785–92

Part III: Alternative Solutions

Chapter 9: The Best Heart-healthy Diet

1. Circulation, 2014; 130: 10–7
2. Lancet Diabetes Endocrinol, 2014; 2: 648–54
3. Am J Clin Nutr, 1995; 61 [6 Suppl]: 1360S–7S
4. N Engl J Med, 2013; 368: 1279–90
5. Diabetes Care, 2013; 36: 3803–11
6. Proc Natl Acad Sci U S A, 2014; 111: 8167–72
7. BMJ, 1996; 313: 775–9
8. Lancet, 2002; 359: 1969–74
9. J Hypertens, 1991; 9: 465–73; J Hypertens, 1992; 10: 195–9
10. Hypertension, 2001; 38: 821–6
11. N Engl J Med, 1987; 316: 235–40
12. BMJ, 1990; 301: 521–3
13. Am J Epidemiol, 1987; 126: 1093–102
14. Ann Med, 2014; 46: 182–7
15. World Rev Nutr Diet, 1990; 62: 120–85
16. Lancet, 1999; 353: 1045–8

17. J Am Coll Cardiol, 2009; 53: 2283–7

18. Cochrane Database Syst Rev, 2007; 3: CD005105

19. Arch Intern Med, 2010; 170: 136–45

20. JAMA, 2007; 297: 969–77

21. J Nutr, 2004; 134: 104–11

22. Circulation, 2013; 128: 337–43

23. Am J Clin Nutr, 2004; 80: 1175–84; J Intern Med, 2005; 258: 153–65

24. J Am Coll Nutr, 1996; 15: 325–39

25. Biomed Pharmacother, 2002; 56: 365–79

26. Arch Intern Med, 2001; 161: 2573–8

27. Perm J, 2011; 15: 19–25

28. Stroke, 2011; 42: 908–12

29. JAMA, 2008; 299: 308–15

30. BMJ, 1995; 310: 693–6

31. Arch Latinoam Nutr, 2004; 54: 380–94

32. J Intern Med, 2009; 266: 248–57

33. Hypertension, 2005; 46: 398–405

34. JAMA, 2007; 298: 49–60

35. Free Radic Biol Med, 2004; 37: 1351–9

36. Circulation, 2007; 116: 2376–82

37. J Am Coll Nutr, 2004; 23: 197–204

38. Nutr Today, 2002; 37: 103–9

39. Med Hypotheses, 2010; 74: 370–3

40. Recent Pat Anticancer Drug Discov, 2012; 7: 14–30

41. Eur J Endocrinol, 2009; 160: 25–31

42. Popul Res Policy Rev, 2013; 32: 325–52

43. BMJ, 2009; 338: b2337

44. FASEB J, 2009; 23: 2412–24

45. www.sciencedaily.com/releases/2011/04/110403090259.htm

46. Br J Diabetes Vasc Dis, 2013; 13: 68–72

47. Br J Pharmacol, 2012; 165: 574–90

48. BMC Med, 2013; 11: 164

49. J Nutr, 2013; 143: 788–94

50. J Nutr, 2010; 141: 56–62

51. Free Radic Res, 2014; 48: 599–606

52. Stroke, 2011; 42: 3190–5

53. BMJ, 2013; 347: f7267

54. Evid Based Complement Alternat Med, Article ID 918384, in press

55. www.sciencedaily.com/releases/2012/03/120326113331.htm

56. Br J Clin Pharmacol, 2013; 75: 677–96

57. CMAJ, 2014; doi: 10.1503/cmaj.131727

58. PLoS One, 2014; 9: e99070

59. FASEB J, 2011; 25: 1793–814

60. Mol Nutr Food Res, 2012; 56: 1106–21

61. Arch Intern Med, 2007; 167: 1730–7

62. Am J Clin Nutr, 2010; 92: 1251–6

63. Am J Clin Nutr, 2006; 84: 762–73

64. N Engl J Med, 1993; 328: 1450–6, 1444–9

65. J Thorac Cardiovasc Surg, 1994; 108: 302–10

66. Lancet, 1991; 337: 1–5

67. Am J Clin Nutr, 1999; 69: 1086–107

68. www.sciencedaily.com/releases/2011/11/111113141254.htm

69. Am J Med, 1995; 98: 485–90

70. Eur Heart J, 2013; 34: 1279–91

71. Parsons WB. *Cholesterol Control Without Diet! The Niacin Solution. Scottsdale*, AZ: Lilac Press, 1998

72. Eur Heart J, 1989; 10: 502–8

73. Ann N Y Acad Sci, 2004; 1033: 79–91

74. Tohoku J Exp Med, 1983; 141 Suppl: 453–63; J Clin Pharmacol, 1990; 30: 596–608

75. Regul Toxicol Pharmacol, 2007; 47: 19–28

76. Am J Cardiol, 1995; 76: 459–62

77. Eur J Clin Nutr, 2012; 66: 411–8

78. Am J Clin Nutr, 2004; 80 [6 Suppl]: 1678S–88S

79. Hypertension, 2014; 64: 897–903

Chapter 10: Proven Alternative Treatments for Heart Disease

1. J Hum Hypertens, 1988; 2: 207–17

2. N Engl J Med, 1978; 298: 1–6

3. Lancet, 2006; 368: 666–78

4. Nutr J, 2009; 8: 5

5. Biol Pharm Bull, 2005; 28: 1208–10

6. Am J Hypertens, 2014; 27: 899–906

7. BMC Cardiovasc Disord, 2008; 8: 13

8. Drugs Exp Clin Res, 2000; 26: 89–93

9. Am Heart J, 2006; 151: 100

10. J Agric Food Chem, 2005; 53: 8106–15

11. Mezger J. *Gesichtete Homöopathische Arzneimittellehre,* 4th edn. Heidelberg: Karl F. Haug Verlag, 1977

12. Maturitas, 2010; 67: 144–50

13. J Clin Epidemiol, 1995; 48: 927–40

14. JAMA, 2013; 309: 1241–50

15. www.poison.org/current/chelationtherapy.htm

16. Br Med J [Clin Res Ed], 1985; 290: 1103–6

17. Auton Neurosci, 2011; 161: 116–20; J Card Fail, 2002; 8: 399–406

18. J Med Food, 2013; 16: 103–11

19. Biotechnol Res Int, 2012; 2012: 976203

20. Natural Med J, 2011; http://naturalmedicinejournal.com/journal/2011–07/ hibiscus–hawthorn–and–heart

21. Bode AM, Dong Z, 'Chapter 7 The Amazing and Mighty Ginger', in Benzie IFF, Wachtel–Galor S, eds. *Herbal Medicine: Biomolecular and Clinical Aspects,* 2nd edn. Boca Raton, FL: CRC Press, 2011

22. Wien Med Wochenschr, 1989; 139: 92–4

23. Int J Cardiol, 1995; 49: 191–9

24. J Tongji Med Univ, 1993; 13: 193–8

25. J Assoc Physicians India, 1989; 37: 323–8

26. J Am Coll Cardiol, 1995; 25: 1076–83

27. Circulation, 1986; 74: 1124–36

28. Cardiovasc Res, 1998; 40: 9–22

29. Circulation, 1990; 82: 2044–51

30. Arzneimittelforschung, 1993; 43: 945–9

31. Am J Cardiol, 1985; 56: 247–51

32. Am J Clin Nutr, 2013; 97: 268–75

33. Planta Med, 1994; 60: 101–5

34. Al–Nimer MSM. 'Evaluation of anti–ischemic therapy in coronary artery disease: a review', in Chaikovsky I, ed. *Coronary Artery Diseases.* InTech: 2012: 177–8; www.intechopen.com

35. Zhonghua Xin Xue Guan Bing Za Zhi, 1990; 18: 155–6, 190

36. Angiology, 1969; 20: 22–6

37. Jpn Heart J, 1990; 31: 829–35

38. Eur Heart J Suppl, 2013; 1 (S2): 124

39. Eur J Clin Pharmacol, 1993; 45: 333–6

40. J Tradit Chin Med, 1986; 6: 235–8

41. J Public Health [Oxf], 2011; 33: 496–502

42. Brain, 2008; 131: 866–76

43. Proc Natl Acad Sci U S A, 2009; 106: 6011–6

44. Stroke, 2007; 38: 1293–7

45. Cochrane Database Syst Rev, 2011; 9: CD008349

46. Top Stroke Rehabil, 2007; 14: 9–22

47. Stroke, 2010; 41: 2044–9

48. CNS Neurosci Ther, 2008; 14: 287–94

49. Weiss RF. *Herbal Medicine*. Gothenburg, Sweden: Ab Arcanum, 1988: 149–51

50. AHZ, 1960; 205: 311–8, 337–58

51. www.vithoulkas.com/en/books–study/online–materia–medica/3812–spartium–scoparium.html

52. Leeser O. *Lehrbuch der Homöopathie, vol 2 (Textbook of Homeopathy)*. Heidelberg: Karl F. Haug Verlag, 1971: 562; AHZ, 1961; 206: 114–5

53. O'Connor J, Bensky D (transl). *Shanghai College of Traditional Medicine: Acupuncture–A Comprehensive Text*. Seattle, WA: Eastland Press, 1981: 252–4

54. Am J Cardiol, 2007; 99: 1726–32

Chapter 11: The Heart–healthy Lifestyle

1. BMJ, 2013; 347: f5577

2. Br J Sports Med, 2014; 48: 239–43

3. Stroke, 2014; 45: 194–9

4. Stroke, 1998; 29: 2049–54

5. Am J Epidemiol, 1996; 143: 860–9

6. Med Sci Sports Exerc, 2000; 32 [9 suppl]: 5498–504

7. J Sports Med Phys Fitness, 2000; 40: 297–302

8. N Engl J Med, 1999; 341: 650–8

9. N Engl J Med, 2002; 5: 347: 716–25

10. Br J Sports Med, 1994; 28: 261–6

11. Metabolism, 1994; 43: 836–41

12. Med Sci Sports Exerc, 1996; 28: 1235–42

13. Int J Obes Relat Metab Disord, 2000; 24: 1303–9

14. Med Sci Sports Exerc, 1998; 30: 152–7

15. Prev Med, 2005; 41: 92–7

16. Med Sci Sports Exerc, 2002; 34: 1468–74

17. Clin J Sport Med, 1997; 7: 28–31

18. Scand J Med Sci Sports, 1996; 6: 222–7

19. Cochrane Database Syst Rev, 2001, 7: CD001256

20. J Am Coll Cardiol, 2013; 62: 709–14

21. J Clin Hypertens [Greenwich], 2007; 9: 800–1; J Altern Complement Med, 2003; 9: 747–54; J Altern Complement Med, 2008; 14: 27–37

22. Ibid.

23. Stroke, 2008; 39: 3185–92

24. Nurs Forum, 1991; 26: 9–16

25. Traumatology, 1999; 5: 1, article 4

26. Explore [NY], 2006; 2: 498–508

Chapter 12: Staying Connected

1. Am J Public Health, 1992; 82: 1089–92

2. Wolf S, Bruhn JG. *The Power of Clan. The Influence of Human Relationships on Heart Disease.* New Brunswick, NJ: Transaction Publishers, 1993

3. Health Soc Work, 2008; 33: 9–21

4. Proc R Soc B, 2010; 277: 529–37

5. Am J Epidemiol, 1979; 109: 186–204; 1988; 128: 370–80

6. PLoS Med, 2010; 7: e1000316

7. Psychosom Med, 2001; 63: 267–72

8. Psychol Aging, 2010; 25: 132–41

9. Soc Sci Med, 2010; 71: 181–6

10. Psychoneuroendocrinology, 2011; 36: 200–9

11. BMC Med, 2014; 12: 42

12. Am J Epidemiol, 1983; 117: 384–96

13. Arch Gen Psychiatry, 2007; 64: 234–40

14. J Biosoc Sci, 2006; 38: 835–42

15. Cancer Prev Res [Phila], 2009; 2: 850–61

16. BBC News, 29 September 2009; http://news.bbc.co.uk/2/hi/health/8279425.stm

17. Epidemiology, 2011; 22: 1–5

18. Psychosom Med, 2001; 63: 273–4

19. Arch Pediatr Adolesc Med, 2006; 160: 805–11

20. Tex Heart Inst J, 2007; 34: 76–9

21. N Engl J Med, 2005; 352: 539–48

22. Stroke, 2007; 38: 993–7

23. J Nerv Ment Dis, 2008; 196: 79–83

24. Altern Ther Health Med, 2006; 12: 26–35

25. Int J Psychiatry Med, 2011; 42: 13–28

26. Explore [NY], 2006; 2: 498–508

27. Am J Cardiol, 2013; 112: 1120–5

28. Dossey L. *The Extraordinary Healing Powers of Ordinary Things.* New York: Harmony Books, 2006

29. Am J Cardiol, 2005; 95: 1060–4

30. Circ Cardiovasc Qual Outcomes, 2012; 5: 750–8

31. Z Psychosom Med Psychother, 2005; 51: 57–80

32. Complement Ther Med, 2007; 15: 157–63

ACKNOWLEDGEMENTS

Every book is a collective activity, and none more so than this one, which bears the silent fingerprints of a raft of people involved with What Doctors Don't Tell You, the publication and website, since its beginnings in 1989.

Much of the information contained in this book represents the best material gathered over the years about heart disease by a number of WDDTY writers and editors, and published in one form or another in our newsletter or magazine, or on our website. They include, chiefly, Bryan Hubbard, Lynne McTaggart and Joanna Evans, but also Dr Harald Gaier – WDDTY's Medical Detective – Tessa Thomas and Kim Wallace. We are also indebted to a number of doctors and practitioners for their help with research and ideas, particularly Dr Patrick Kingsley and Dr John Mansfield.

Thanks are particularly due to Alison Rose Levy, who was involved in the initial assembly of this material; Sharyn Wong, WDDTY's production editor, for copyediting the manuscript and cross-checking the facts and hundreds of references cited in this book; and Jo Evans, for some last minute edits and additions.

The entire staff at Hay House has our deep gratitude for their enthusiastic and courageous embracing of this project, but most particularly Reid Tracy, Michelle Pilley, Julie Oughton and Jo Burgess. We are also indebted to Bob Saxton for his careful copyediting and suggestions, which improved the manuscript in countless ways.

Finally we are grateful to the other members of WDDTY's indefatigable UK team, who add to its mission in countless ways, including John Clement, Jimmy Egerton, Trevor Jayakody, Oliver Kemp, Alice Rhodes, Paul Barrett, Mark Jones, Bruce Sawford and our teams at Comag and Esco who handle distribution and subscriptions.

Two others are responsible, in a sense, for the birth of this manuscript. As a young journalist, one of us (Lynne) was privileged to edit the work of Dr Robert Mendelsohn, whose prescient views about medicine initially influenced both of us. We were also extremely fortunate to have come across Dr Stephen Davies, the nutritional pioneer who not only successfully treated Lynne's condition but also helped us to view disease and the means to treat it in a completely new light. They were the midwives who gave birth to what has become a major focus of our journalistic work - what we have come believe is the biggest, most important story of all.

||||||||||||||||||||||||||||||||||||||||||||||||

INDEX

beans, pulses and legumes 39, 48, 138,
140, 145, 147–8, 151, 154, 204
kidney 141, 145, 204
soya 7, 141, 145
beetroot juice 154
beliefs 199
belonging, sense of 189–202
Benecol 51–3
Berberis vulgaris 171
bereavement 196, 198

HAY HOUSE

Look within

Join the conversation about latest products,
events, exclusive offers and more.

 Hay House UK

 @HayHouseUK

 @hayhouseuk

♥ healyourlife.com

We'd love to hear from you!